Yoga

How to Use Yoga to Relieve Stress, Build Wealth, and Achieve Harmony!

(The Philosophy of Yoga Sutras and the Secret of Sleep Meditation and Deep Relaxation With Yoga Nidra)

Deborah Lacerda

Published by Rob Miles

Deborah Lacerda

All Rights Reserved

Yoga: How to Use Yoga to Relieve Stress, Build Wealth, and Achieve Harmony! (The Philosophy of Yoga Sutras and the Secret of Sleep Meditation and Deep Relaxation With Yoga Nidra)

ISBN 978-1-989990-55-1

Legal & Disclaimer

The information contained in this book is not designed to replace or take the place of any form of medicine or professional medical advice. The information in this book has been provided for educational and entertainment purposes only.

The information contained in this book has been compiled from sources deemed reliable, and it is accurate to the best of the Author's knowledge; however, the Author cannot guarantee its accuracy and validity and cannot be held liable for any errors or omissions. Changes are periodically made to this book. You must consult your doctor or get professional medical advice before using any of the suggested remedies, techniques, or information in this book.

Table of Contents

INTRODUCTION

Yoga is more than merely an exercise. Although it includes moves to stretch, realign, and animate the body, to think that it is merely a physical experience, renders the prospective student of Yoga at a disadvantage. To truly understand Yoga, one must understand the extent of human composition. Living organisms manifest from its surroundings much like ice, from water. Ice emerges from water when conditions are right, and return to water when conditions cease to exist. Human beings are no different.

Those conditions are influenced by everything - tangible and intangible, that surrounds us. Even a waxing or waning moon holds sway over our mental state, psychology, and ultimately, our state of balance. When these forces, beyond our control, alter our balance we feel it in different ways. It can result in transient ailments, aches, and pains; diminished moods and depressed motivation; or, sadness, worry, and anger.

Technology has given us the ability to create potions and concoctions that seek to return us to that state of balance. However, they only address the symptoms that bother us, not the imbalance that plagues us. Due to those influences, the balance that renders us peaceful is sometimes stressed and stretched until everything from our metabolism, to our physiology, and mental acuity are imperiled.

When balance is restored, the body returns to peace and we feel good once more. We make better decisions when we are at peace. When at peace, we are more efficient at extracting nutrients from the food we eat, we are happier and more productive. At the point of balance, all is well within us.

To put it in binary terms, on one side you have the sum of various forces that alters our balance. On the other side, you have the sum of practices that realign and neutralize the chaos those forces enacted upon us. The latter of the two sides in this binary illustration is Yoga.

Yoga is an ancient practice dating back more than five thousand years. It was developed throughout generations by Vedic scholars in, what is now, the northern provinces of India. The doctors, then, knew that everything is connected. Everything from the direction of the wind, to the location of the celestial bodies, and the content of our meals, exacted a net effect on our balance. As they developed their understanding, the layers of Yoga developed further.

Western medicine is not solely the realm of a GP doctor. It consists of all the different professional branches ranging from neurology to podiatry, and psychology to physiotherapy. There are many branches under one overarching umbrella, we call medicine. Yoga is the same way. It is not just the twisting and contorting of the body, it includes how one breathes, the way one eats, how one sleeps, and even how one thinks. All of it comes under one overarching umbrella, the ancients called Yoga.

Yoga consists of eight parts. The part concerning postures is the one most people, today, associate with Yoga. But Yoga is much more than that. The limb of Yoga that focuses on postures is called the Asana in the Sanskrit language. The seven other parts include Niyama, Yama, Pranayama, Pratyahara, Dharana, Dhyana, and Samadhi.

When these eight limbs of Yoga are practiced, they serve to rebalance the effect that results from the forces of the Universe tugging at our existence and open the path to enlightenment.A life lived outside the balance of peace is miserable and unproductive. But a life that includes all or some of the eight limbs of Yoga is naturally at peace.

Some of the most powerful and effective world-class athletes use Yoga as the core of their training. It has proven effective in high-impact training and provides the balance and conditioning that athletes need to be competitive and excel at their chosen sport. The same can be said for professional dancers and martial arts fighters.

The realignment of one's life by the practice of Yoga can bring about a deeper understanding of purpose. It has the effect of elevating one's state of being and state of mind. The components that align posture, move the muscles and skeletal structure back to the way millions of years of evolution designed them to be. In its optimal state, the human body is a work of art – perfect in its balance. It allows the uninterrupted flow of fluids, the unimpeded exchange of gases, and the smooth transition of nutrients and waste. Blockages of liquids, solids, and gasses are removed and shunted away, resulting in a comfortable body and neutral chemistry that otherwise would not exist.

When good posture is combined with abstinence and observance, it elevates the mind, to be free from the drag of poor habits and the distraction of primal sensations. When meditation and concentration are added to the mix, the human experience transcends the bounds of physical limitations. We may seem to be only flesh and bone, but Yoga has the power to unleash the full potential that lays within, to reveal we are more.

As powerful as Yoga is, it needs to be absorbed not mimicked, practiced more than it is preached, and included in every facet of one's life, not just the hours spent at the Yoga studio. Do not rush into it. Take the time to organically absorb it. Each step, when done correctly, will flow into the next.

CHAPTER 1: SIGNIFICANCE OF YOGA MUDRAS

BENEFITS AND MEANINGS

Significance of yoga mudras

Entirely distinct and based on the principle of Ayurveda, yoga mudras are understood as a healing modality. The Sanskrit word mudra is translated as a gesture. A mudra may involve the whole body or could be a simple hand position. Mudras used in combination with yoga breathing exercises enliven the flow of prana in the body, thereby energizing different parts of the body.

How do yoga mudras work?

Diseases are caused due to an imbalance in the body, which in turn is caused by lack or excess of any of the five elements.

Our fingers have the characteristics of these elements and each of these five elements serves a specific and important function within the body. The fingers are essentially electrical circuits. The use of mudras adjusts the flow of energy - affecting the balance of air, fire, water, earth, ether - and facilitate healing.

Mudras create a subtle connection with the instinctual patterns in the brain and influence the unconscious reflexes in these areas. The internal energy is, in turn, balanced and redirected, affecting change in the sensory organs, glands, veins and tendons.

Yoga mudras are practiced sitting simply cross-legged, in Vajrasana or in the lotus posture, or even by sitting comfortably on a chair. Ideally, Ujjai breathing is done when practicing most mudras.

In each yoga mudra, take at least twelve breaths and closely observe the flow of energy in the body.

Chin Mudra

Hold the thumb and index finger together lightly while extending the remaining three fingers.

The thumb and index finger need only touch together, without exerting any pressure.

Keep the three extended fingers as straight as possible.

The hands can then be placed on the thighs, facing upwards.

Now, observe the flow of breath and its effect.

Benefits of Chin Mudra

•Better retention and concentration power

•Improves sleep pattern

•Increases energy in the body

•Alleviates lower backache

Chinmaya Mudra

In this mudra, the thumb and forefinger form a ring and the three remaining fingers are curled into the palms of the hands.

Again, the hands are placed on the thighs with palms facing upwards and deep comfortable Ujjai breaths are taken.

Once more, observe the flow of breath and its effect.

Benefits of Chinmaya Mudra

•Improves flow of energy in the body

•Stimulates digestion

Adi Mudra

In Adi Mudra, the thumb is placed at the base of the small finger and the remaining fingers curl over the thumb, forming a light fist.

The palms are again placed facing upwards on the thighs and the breathing repeated.

Benefits of Adi Mudra

•Relaxes the nervous system

•Helps reduce snoring

•Improves the flow of oxygen to the head

•Increases capacity of the lungs

Brahma Mudra

Here both hands are placed in Adi Mudra, then with the knuckles of both hands together, the hands facing upward are placed at the navel area and the flow of breath continued.

Feeling held back due to a physical ailment? Are emotions taking a toll on your personal and work life? Fill in the form below to learn more about how yoga can aide you in overcoming issues naturally with minimum lifestyle changes.

Mudras is considered to be the world's oldest holistic healing system and often described as yoga's 'sister science' - disease is the result of an imbalance in our body caused by a deficiency or an excess one of the five key elements: space, air, fire, water and earth. Each of these is said to play a specific role within the body and are represented by the five fingers:

The thumb - fire

The forefinger - wind

The middle finger - ether (or space)

The ring finger - earth

The little finger - water

The fingers essentially act as electrical circuits and the use of mudras adjust the flow of energy which balance these various elements and accommodate healing.

The fingers essentially act as electrical circuits and the use of mudras adjust the flow of energy which balance these various elements and accommodate healing.

Benefits of Mudras

The mudras benefit the bio magnetic fields, psyche, body, and mind in many waysc Some of the benefits of mudras are as follows:

The mudras clear the psychic centers and subtle channels in the body This allows the life force to flow freely to the various parts of the bodyt

The mudras purify the body's bio magnetic field and shield it from negative forcesd

Purpose of Mudras

The purpose of mudras is to bring about a complete regeneration and transformation of the body-mind principle and an expansion of the consciousnessn However, make sure that you consult your doctor before practicing yoga mudraso This is because certain conditions like diabetes can worsen with the practice of yoga mudras.

Chapter 2: Holistically Speaking

If you consider the body and the way that energy flows through it, acupuncturists are always telling patients about the flow of yin and yang through the body. In yoga, this is translated a little differently in that you have something that is called chakras. These are points in the body where energy can get blocked and the exercises that you do during yoga sessions help you to free these up, so that your body is in perfect harmony with your mind. You don't get much more holistic than that.

You may have images of people sitting in very awkward positions, but you really don't have to do that if you find it too difficult. What you do need to understand is the role of the chakras and how the different exercises that you do during typical yoga classes help you holistically to feel more at peace with yourself.

If you want to make the most of yoga, you really would do well to go to a class because qualified instructors will know which exercises will benefit the part of the body which you feel needs improvement. For many people, yoga is a way of finding answers to problems that are more lasting than fads such as diets and exercise that wears them out and doesn't seem to help at all. The problem is that you can overdo it and yoga isn't about how much you hurt. It's about how much you heal and there lies the difference.

In conjunction with the exercises shown in the following chapters, you will need to be sensible about your diet and make sure that you include a good variety of foods and that you avoid those foods which make you feel bloated and uncomfortable. Never perform yoga with a full stomach because that isn't the ideal at all. In fact, yoga instructors recommend that you perform your yoga before mail meals with a couple of hours between doing your yoga and eating – thus giving the body a good chance to feel great. What you can have during your yoga sessions is water.

Though you may consider that you drink sufficient water in tea and coffee, you may be fooling yourself. Tea and coffee are stimulants and do not act in the same way as regular water. You have to try and get over this feeling that you don't like water, because this will help you considerably to get rid of aches and pains and help your body to become more flexible.

Do you need props?

Not many. In short, it isn't about the kit you have. It's about having a mat and a small cushion, as well as wearing comfortable clothing that does not constrict your body. There are those who spend a lot of money on kit, but you really don't need it and it's not what yoga is all about. It's a holistic way to help your body to recover from the stresses and strains of life without pushing it past acceptable limits.

Unlike other sports, you are not going to be expected to push your limits. You will not be asked to do things that you find difficult and if you are, you are encouraged to ease yourself into the exercises, because yoga is not about suffering. It's about alleviating suffering and is a discipline rather than a sport.

How can you not feel good about greeting the sun? As you read through the yoga exercises and learn how they are done, remember that the most holistic exercise that is practiced by yoga students is the sun salutation. It energizes you. It stretches you and then gently relaxes you and it is this exercise that you will number among your favorites because it's invigorating.

As you practice yoga, you also need to learn all about the benefits of meditation as hand in hand with exercises, this is valuable and helps you to slow down your way of thinking so that you can gain the most insight from your experience. Yoga meditation is performed by performing breathing exercises and these form a very important part of yoga exercises as well, with the air that you breathe in and out helping you to measure your movements and go with the flow.

Yoga is a wonderful addition to your life. It takes time to perfect the movements, but once you do, even at beginner level, you will begin to embrace the holistic experience and feel it start to make you feel whole. It will change your attitude to life. It will help you to see your lifestyle in another light – one that encourages the right kinds of food and gentleness to yourself. You are precious and with practice, you will heal your mind, lose weight and feel so much better for your experience.

CHAPTER 3: HOW I CAME TO LEARN ABOUT FOOT YOGA

I have been teaching yoga for over 13 years. In the thousands of yoga classes that I have taught, I've seen a lot of feet. From healthy feet to feet that barely want to support a person. I've seen a wide variety of feet with high arches, no arches, bunions, hammer toes, misshaped toes, toes so squished together you can't separate them, and so on. All of these feet have a story to tell about their owner, & if they could talk, your feet would tell your story, too.

In yoga class, we usually take our socks off. Right away, I can start to see how much care someone takes of their feet. If a student dislikes even looking at their feet, then this is often a sign that they have been neglecting their feet or that they are unhappy with their feet. I often hear comments about needing a pedicure just to make your feet presentable.

Overall, there seems to be a common dislike of our feet. Exercise: Take a moment, right now, and just look at your feet. What do you notice? What do you like? What do you dislike? What do you feel in your feet? What do you feel about your feet? Just start with a visual examination of your feet & see where it takes you.

What's interesting to me is that when you neglect a part of your body, in this case, your feet, then that part of your body will start to talk to you in one form or another. If you don't listen to what your feet are saying, then that discussion will get louder and louder until you have no choice but to pay attention. All of a sudden, it hurts to walk or even just stand and you are left with little choice but to do something that will help your feet.

So often, what happens is that you have developed a habit of mistreating your feet. You're constantly putting them into shoes that are too small or too narrow to allow them to form their natural state, for

20

example. This can result in misshapen toes that just don't feel good. Or maybe you grip with your toes out of anxiety or habit, and this can contribute to having hammer toes. Putting too much pressure on one part of your foot can contribute to bunions. Not exercising or stretching the foot can lead to Plantar Fasciitis. All of these foot conditions can be painful if left untreated.

Over my years of teaching classes, I've learned several ways to work with feet so that they simply feel better. I've given the following simple exercises to so many people. Often, those same people come back to me, sometimes months later, and say how much better their feet feel. These simple exercises were so helpful to them that they made a point to thank me. This tells me that these exercises can work for many people. These exercises are free and easy to do. Except for a couple, you don't even need any equipment. They are easy to practice and they work so well. While I won't promise that these exercises and tricks will fix all of your foot problems, I will tell you that your feet can feel better.Of course, how much better depends on a lot of variables, but when your feet hurt, even feeling a little bit better is a blessing. And...when your feet feel better, then the rest of your body feels better. So, why are you waiting? Take better care of your feet today!

FootStretches

If you've ever been to an exercise class (yoga or any other type), then you've been taken through stretches for the body. These stretches are usually designed to increase flexibility and blood flow to the various parts of your body and to keep you from getting any injuries. In general, these stretches you're doing keep your body healthier.

Now, think back to the last exercise class that you did. Were there any foot stretches? Did the instructor say anything about how to make your feet healthier? Chances are the answer to those questions is a "no". Usually, whether in a formal class, book, or video, the focus is on the larger muscles in the body. We stretch our arms, legs, backs, sides of the body, etc., but we tend to overlook the feet. It's time to change that.

There are over 100 muscles, ligaments, and tendons in a foot. There are also 33 joints. That's a lot of tissue in a small, compact space, and a lot of places where the foot can bend. It's no wonder that when we consistently put our feet in shoes that don't fit well or are too small, that our amazing feet lose the ability to perform as they were designed to do.

These muscles, ligaments, and tendons need to be stretched just like other parts of your body, and all your joints will be a part of this. If you've ever spent any time stretching, then you know how good it can feel to do so. Well, the same can be said about stretching a foot. It will feel so good, and you'll wonder why you haven't done these stretches before.

Now, the first thing that you need to do is take off your shoes. I know for some of us, that's a huge step. I know people who only take off their shoes to bathe or go to bed. They absolutely refuse to go barefoot for any length of time. This saddens me because wearing shoes constantly will slowly weaken the foot. The foot begins to rely on the shoe for support and the muscles will be used less. This can create a downward cycle where your feet become weaker from shoes and so you wear your shoes more.

We'll get back to this later, but for now, take off your shoes. Start by just looking at your feet. Notice any changes that have happened. Maybe you have some bunions or hammer toes. Maybe your toes are crowded from narrow shoes. Are your arches high or low? Do you even have arches in your feet? Practice a little awareness now to give yourself a good baseline of what your feet are like. Maybe even take a picture so that you don't have to rely on your memory. That way, when you look at them in a week, month or year, you'll notice any changes that you see.

A foot can move in multiple ways. I like to think that they are remarkable feats of engineering. Spend a moment just wiggling your toes, pointing and flexing your foot, turning it from side to side. Notice the various ways that your foot can naturally move. If you're finding that your range of movement is limited, then these stretches and exercises can help you to regain your mobility. It just takes a little time and patience.

CHAPTER 4

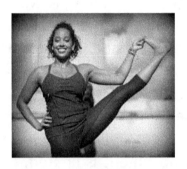

To be able to teach yoga in a professional capacity it is important that you understand anatomy and physiology. You need to know the areas of the body which are affected by individual yoga postures so you can discuss benefits and contraindications.

The human body is ingenious. In essence, it is an incredible array of components which are all neatly assembled together. We have muscles, nerves vital organs, glands, circulatory systems and the skeleton.

The skeleton has 214 bones, let's take a closer look at the various parts of the skeleton:

Axial   skeleton
Bones within the axial skeleton include: the skull, ribs, sternum (breastbone) vertebral column (backbone).

Appendicular   skeleton
This part of the skeleton includes: the limbs, pelvic girdle and shoulder girdle. Bones are classified in relation to their shape and formations:

Short bones - include those found in the wrists

Long bones-include those found in the fingers

Flat bones-include those found in the shoulder blades/ skull Sesamoid bones-those bones developed in the tendons i.e. the kneecap Irregular bones -found within the vertebrae or the face

Let's take a close look at the skull. There are two main parts of the skull-the face and the cranium. There are 14 bones in the face:

2nasalbones
2Palatinebones
2Lacrimabones
2Zygomaticbones
1Vome
2inferiorturbinatebones
 Maxillae
1 mandible

The cranium has eight bones:

1occipitalbone
2parietalbones
1frontalbone
2temporalbones
1Sphenoidbone
1 Ethmoid bone

The vertebral column has 33 bones (or sometimes 34). Each individual bone is known as a vertebra. The top 7 vertebrae are known as the cervical vertebrae and it is the two top cervical vertebrae that afford the movement of the neck. The first cervical vertebrae are known as the atlas and the second is known as the axis. The top two vertebrae form the Atlanto-Axial joint.

Then, there are 12 thoracic vertebrae Moving further down, there are 5 lumbar vertebrae.

Then, 5 sacral vertebrae and these form the sacrum. In adults, these 5 vertebrae are   fused.

Lastly, we have the tailbone-known as the coccyx and these have 4 or 5 Coccygeal vertebrate. As in the say cruel region, the vertebrae of the coccyx are fused in adults.

Thoracic   cage

The thoracic cage includes the 12 thoracic vertebrae as listed above and then 12 pairs of ribs at the sides and the sternum at the front.

At the top of the thoracic cage there are 7 pairs of true ribs, then just below, there are 3 pairs of false ribs and 2 pairs of floating ribs. The pairs of true ribs attached directly to the sternum and the 3 pairs of false ribs are connected indirectly by way of an attachment of cartilage that extends from each of the ribs to the rib above. Finally, the 2 pairs of floating ribs are not attached to the sternum at all.

Above the thoracic cage, there is the shoulder girdle: Left and right clavicle (collarbones) Left and right scapula (shoulder blades)

A small bone known as the hyoid bone sits in isolation at the front of the throat.

The arms are attached to each side of the shoulder girdle. The bone nearest to the shoulder is the humorous and this is the bone of the upper arm. In the lower part of the arm, the two bones which are placed side-by-side are known as the radius and ulna.

The wrist and hand
There are 8 bones which make up the carpus:

Navicular (scaphoid) Lunate (Semilunar) Triquetral
Pisiform
Trapezium

Trapezoid
Capitate
Hamate

There are 5 metacarpals which make up the bones between the fingers and wrist and then 14 phalanges which form the 4 fingers and thumb.

Then, moving back to the main skeletal area, there is the pelvic girdle and this consists of the 5th lumbar vertebrae, the sacrum, and the coccyx at the back. There are also 2 innominate bones which circle the remainder.

Moving down to the leg bones: Femur (thighbone)
Patella(kneecap)
Tibia(shinbone)
Fibula (alongside the tibia)

The bones of the foot are as follows: There are 7 bones which make up the tarsus including:

Calcaneum(Heel)Talus
Navicular

Cuboid

3 x Cuneiforms

5 metatarsals and 14 phalanges form the toes.

Now let's take a look at the joints of the skeleton. A joint (also known as articulation) is the union of 2 or more bones.

There are three main types of joints:

Fibrous

Cartilaginous Synovial

They vary considerably as regards movement and are classified as follows:

Immovable

Slightly movable Freely movable

Immovable fibrous joints. These are fixed joints where no movement is allowed at all. These are the joints of the flat bones of the skull and, the teeth sockets.

Cartilaginous joints are slightly movable and the surface of the joints are separated by substance such as cartilage. Think of the inter-vertebral joints of the vertebrae column and the fibro-cartilage discs.

Synovial joints are freely movable and the end of the bones are covered by hyaline cartilage. Ligaments serve to bind to the bones together and synovial fluid fills the joint cavity and this is enclosed by fibrous tissue.

The following is a list of the varieties are synovial joints and examples of where they might be found:

Gliding – small bones within the carpus
Ball and socket - hip joint
Hinge - elbow joint
Condyloid - wrist joint
Pivot - atlantoaxial joint
Saddle - the joint existing between the trapezium and the first metacarpal bone

Skeletal   muscles
Skeletal muscles are responsible for voluntary movement under the control of the nervous system.

Muscles produce movement as a result of their connection with bones, ligaments, cartilage, fasciae and skin. Typically, these muscles are attached at 2 points – a fixed point which is known as the origin and 1 movable point known as the insertion. Usually, the 2 points are at a distance from each other and the muscle function stands across several joints. At the points of insertion and origin, there are attachments which have become toughened - these are known as the tendons and these are inserted in the bones and other structures.

The muscles of the skeleton work in groups. Try to imagine each group working in opposition to another group i.e. the antagonist. A perfect example of this, are the biceps and triceps. The nervous system stimulates the bicep muscle which contracts i.e. shortens and thickens and the point of insertion in the radius draws towards its origin point in the shoulder joint. This is the process to bend the arm. To reverse this movement, the biceps give way to the opposing pull of the triceps as they contract.

So, the biceps work in opposition to the triceps and of course, vice versa.

The muscles have varying functions and have been classified in accordance. There are extensors responsible for extending and straightening of any limb. For bending the limb, there are antagonist known as flexors, there are also abductors and adductors and pronators and supinator's.

The following is an example of the origin: O, the insertion: I and action of the sterno-mastoid: As a yoga instructor, you must understand how the muscles of the body works and the relevance to the yoga postures.

Sterno-mastoid

The origin is the sternum and clavicle The insertion is the mastoid process of the temporal bone The action is to be able to turn and flex the neck

Self-Assessment Tasks

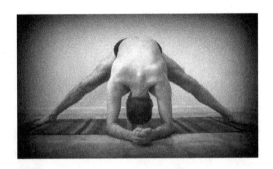

Task:
How many bones are there in the skeleton?

Task:
State the names of the bones within the Axial   skeleton

Task:
State the three main types of joints

Task:
What are skeletal muscles responsible for?

Task:
How many bones make up the carpus?
Please note that these self-assessment tasks are to ensure your understanding of the information within each module. As

such, do not submit them for review with KEW Training Academy.

CHAPTER 5: YOGA FOR ARTHRITIS

Shoulder Pain

A lot of people walk around with the weight of the world on their shoulders. If you have arthritis pain in your shoulders, the tension so many people hold there might be making things even worse. One of the best tonics for shoulder tension is a massage, but many people with arthritis hesitate to get one because massages can be too painful for inflamed joints and the surrounding tissues.

Sitting behind a computer all day is especially bad for shoulder pain and arthritis because slouching over the computer creates more tension, reduces proper blood flow, and can ruin the alignment of your joints.

The poses in this section will help you to release that tension and bring a gentle stretch to sore, inflamed muscles. Building strength in the muscles of your neck and back will also help take some of the pressure off your shoulders. Regularly doing these stretches will help your joints become more flexible and give you some all-natural tools for treating and preventing pain.

Eagle Arms

Sanskrit name: Garudasana

Eagle Arms is a simple pose you can add to other poses, like Chair Pose or Easy Pose, to enhance the shoulder stretch. Eagle Arms is ideal for when you've been sitting behind a desk all day because it also opens up the upper back and forces you to sit up straight, rather than slouch. Don't forget to do both sides, to keep things balanced.

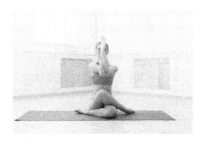

Instructions

Stretch your arms out in front of you and make sure your shoulders are relaxed. Don't allow them to creep up towards your ears.

Cross your left elbow over your right elbow and lift your forearms up towards your face at a 90-degree angle.

Turn your arms inward and try to touch your palms together.

Lift your arms up towards your face to the degree of your comfort. You should feel a stretch across your shoulders and upper back, but if there is any pain, stop immediately.

Hold the pose for 10 breaths, or as long as you can. Don't worry if your form is not perfect, as long as the stretching sensation is comfortable.

Repeat on the other side, crossing your right arm over the left this time.

Thread the Needle

Sanskrit name: Sucirandhrasana

Thread the Needle Pose is a powerful shoulder stretch. It also opens up the chest, which corrects the harmful effects of poor posture on your neck, upper back, and shoulders.

Thread the Needle is not just a great stretch for the shoulders, back, and chest, it's also deeply calming for the central nervous system, which helps to reduce stress and manage pain. Thread the Needle is ideal any time you need a five-minute break, or when arthritis pain and stress are keeping you up at night. If you're finding your arthritis pain hard to manage, a few deep breaths in this pose can have a calming effect, while taking your mind off of the pain.

As well as stretching and aligning your upper body, Thread the Needle is also a twist posture. Twists are said to literally wring out your organs, releasing toxins and stimulating your digestive system. Many people with rheumatoid arthritis end up having to take heavy duty painkillers. This pose could be a great addition to your day to help deal with the digestive side effects of painkiller use.

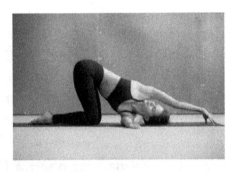

Instructions

Assume tabletop position, on your hands and knees.

Reach your right arm upwards towards the sky, opening your entire side body. Make sure your shoulders are stacked on top of each other, as if you were in side plank, and reach high to open up your chest.

42

Turn and thread your right arm under your left shoulder and inch it forward under your body until your right cheek and right shoulder are resting on the earth.

Scan your body to ensure you are holding no tension in your lower back, buttocks, or neck.

Take 10 deep breaths, or as many are needed to feel relief coming to your shoulders.

Repeat on the other side.

Props

Tabletop position requires you to rest on your knees. If you have sensitive knees, try putting a towel under them to take some of the pressure off. It's also recommended that you use a thicker mat if you have knee pain.

Modifications

If you are pregnant or have severe arthritic knee or wrist pain, you can practice this pose standing up against the wall instead.

Low Lunge Twist Pose

Sanskrit name: Parivrtta Sanchalasana

Low Lunge Twist will help you to open the shoulders, chest, and hips. It will also help to develop strength and flexibility in your shoulders. However, this pose is slightly more advanced and should not be the first pose you do during your practice if you are dealing with shoulder pain. Work your way up to this pose instead, and don't continue if you feel any shooting pains.

Like Thread the Needle, Low Lunge Twist also offers the gentle twisting element that provides the detoxification and relaxation that is so calming for the digestive system, great for those on heavy medications and painkillers.

Interested in the spiritual side of yoga? This pose is said to stimulate energy and open up the heart chakra.

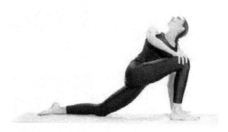

Instructions

Begin in lunge pose with your right leg forward and bent at a 90-degree angle.

Lower your left knee to the ground.

Slowly twist your entire upper body to the right.

From here, you can put your left hand down on the ground and rest your right hand on your knee or lift your right arm skywards.

Take at least five breaths, or rest here as long as needed.

Switch sides and repeat. You can transition through Downward Dog if desired.

Props

This pose calls for you to rest on your knees, so you might want a towel or thicker mat to prevent putting too much pressure on your knees. You can also purchase non-slip gel knee pads made specifically for yoga for around $15.00.

If your shoulders are too tight for your hand to reach the ground, try putting a yoga block beneath your hand.

Modifications

If you are not comfortable putting pressure on your shoulders in this pose, you may add a balancing element, which will make the pose slightly more difficult but will protect your shoulders. Instead of resting on your hand, bring your hands together in prayer pose and rest the back of your left arm on the outside of your right leg.

Cow Face Pose

Sanskrit name: Gomukhasana

Cow Face Pose brings flexibility and strength to the back and shoulders, helping to reduce soreness. It also stretches out your hips. Cow Face Pose can be pretty intense on your shoulders and hips, but if you find it's too much, don't worry. Props can be used to make it much easier. Remember, strength and flexibility come with repetition, so perform the pose only to the degree that it is comfortable.

From a spiritual perspective, this pose opens the heart and sacral chakra.

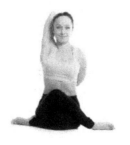

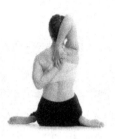

Instructions

Begin seated on the ground. Cross your right leg over your left with your right knee on top of your left knee. Bend your lower legs towards your body so they cross at the knee, and the opposite foot is on either side of your body with the sole facing towards you.

Bend your right arm behind you and inch your hand up the center of your back.

Bend your left arm over your left shoulder and inch your left hand down the center of your back.

Try to touch your hands together, or better yet, grasp each other.

Breathe in this pose for about a minute, then switch sides.

Props

If you are not able to touch your hands together, loop a yoga strap or hand towel between your hands, and grasp that instead.

Modifications

The hip stretch this pose delivers is intense, which is a good thing, but might be too much if you're dealing with a hip injury or arthritis pain. Instead, you can skip the leg posture and focus on the shoulder stretch. Perform the arm posture while sitting erect in a chair, or on a meditation cushion.

Bharadvaja's Twist

Sanskrit name: Bharadvajasana

This pose is named for Bharadvaja, a legendary seer in Hindu tradition. This pose is just as powerful as the seer!

Bharadvaja's Twist brings all the benefits of a twist while broadening your chest and opening your shoulders. It also forces you to sit up straight and brings some much-needed tension relief to your spine. This deeply grounding and relaxing pose is perfect to do before bed.

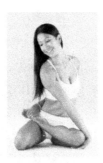

Instructions

Begin seated upright on the floor with your legs out in front of you.

Swing your legs to the right so that both feet are sitting on the outside of your right hip. Then lift your left foot up and move it into the crease of your right hip.

Twist your entire upper body to the left, moving your left hand around your back to grasp your left foot.

Use your right arm to encourage the twist by pressing against your left leg.

Inhale deeply to feel the chest and shoulders opening. Breathe in this pose for 30 seconds to one minute.

Slowly unwind from the pose and repeat on the other side.

Props

If you cannot reach your foot, loop a yoga strap over your foot and grasp it with the appropriate hand.

Modifications

Instead of doing this pose on the ground and moving your foot into your hip arch, you can drop this part of the pose. Sit upright in a chair and twist to the right, grasping the back of the chair for as much leverage as you need. Repeat on the other side.

Standing Forward Fold with Hand Clasp

Sanskrit name: Uttānāsana

Forward folds are soothing poses that help to release stress from the neck and shoulders. If you're holding tension in this area, it's probably making your arthritis pain even worse. This particular fold adds in the hand clasp modification to create even more of a stretch for your shoulders. Standing Forward Fold is also great for insomnia, sore hamstrings, and calming the central nervous system.

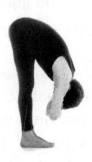

Instructions

Begin standing upright in Mountain Pose.

Exhale as you bend at the hips and allow your head and arms to dangle towards the ground, relaxing your neck. If you like, you can grasp your elbows with your hands to help open the shoulders.

Breath in this pose for as long as you need to relax and feel your shoulders and neck release tension.

Variation for a more challenging pose

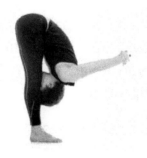

Instructions

Begin standing upright in Mountain Pose. Clasp your hands behind your back and pull them downwards, forcing your back to arch and your chest to open. Inhale deeply.

Exhale as you bend at the hips and allow your head to dangle towards the ground, relaxing your neck. Lift your clasped hands over your head to feel the shoulder stretch.

Breath in this pose for as long as you need to relax and feel your shoulders and neck release tension.

Modifications

If you have knee pain or tight hamstrings, bend your knees until your chest is resting against your thighs. This will create a more relaxing posture.

Reverse Prayer Hands

Sanskrit name: Pashchima Namaskarasana

Reverse Prayer Hands delivers an intense stretch that isn't accessible for many people, even those you don't have arthritis. However, it is a powerful pose to have in your arthritis tool box if you're capable of working your way up to it.

This may be an intermediate pose, but there's lots of good news too! Reverse Prayer Hands brings tons of relief to sore wrists and fingers, spots often hit hard by arthritis that few exercises other than yoga can help. Not only does it open the chest and upper back, it also opens the heart chakra while correcting your posture.

Once you master this pose, you can add it into virtually any other posture. Add Reverse Prayer Hands to lunges, Warrior II, Easy Pose, forward folds, and more!

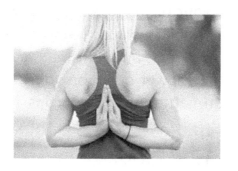

Instructions

Stand upright in Mountain Pose.

Stretch your arms behind you and arch your back.

Point your fingertips upwards and bring your hands together against your back.

The goal is to bring your palms together as if you were praying and to move your hands up to the center of your back, ideally between the shoulder blades.

Breathe and hold the posture as long as needed.

Modifications

Getting your palms to touch and move up to your shoulder blades just isn't going to be possible right away. Instead, start with your hands lower down on your back and focus on getting your fingertips to touch first.

If even that is too intense, lay one hand on your lower back and the other on top. Inhale to open your chest.

Chapter 6: How Yoga Makes You Feel Slim

And Sexier

Stand in front of a full length mirror and stand how you normally do. You probably have bad habits. Your shoulders may be rounded and perhaps you slouch a little. Stand naturally because what you are trying to see is how you are now. Your body may not be that fit and perhaps you don't like what you see. Yoga makes you feel slimmer and sexier because after regular yoga sessions you don't slouch anymore and the way in which you move is so much sexier, being conscious of your movements and also being aware of your breathing method. You will slim down because some of the exercises suggested are aimed at helping to firm up those curves, but what I want you to do now is a simple exercise in front of the mirror which will demonstrate to you how much taller and how much sexier you can look when you practice yoga regularly.

The Talasana Pose

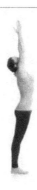

Don't worry. We don't expect you to get this right first time, but it's used in this chapter to demonstrate how sexy and slim you can look by doing the right kind of poses. Yoga poses encourage great posture. You remember how your parents used to tell you to stand straight and hold your shoulders back? Well they did have some point to what they were asking you to do. You may have hated it at the time, but good habits like these help you to grow up standing straight and proud and they weren't just saying it to annoy you. Try this exercise on a mat in the same room where you have the mirror because we want you to look into the mirror at the end of the exercise. You will see a marked difference once you have practiced the Talasana pose a few times.

Stand straight with your feet together, your back straight and make sure that your arms are straight and by your sides with your palms facing your body. Breathe in through the nose, breathe out through the nose. There's a chapter on breathing later on in the book, but for now this is all you need to know.

Inhale deeply and move your arms to straight above your head. Imagine that you are reaching for something high above you. Stretch your fingers as much as you can and, without taking the soles of your feet off the carpet, feel your fingers stretch into the air. Bend your hands back so that the palms of your hands are facing toward the ceiling.

Now lift your ankles from the mat and feel the whole body stretch up to the sky, balancing on your toes for a few moments. On the exhale, bring your arms down slowly, put your whole foot back on the mat and come to the original position. The first time, it's unlikely that you got the breathing right because you were pausing to see what to do next. Now inhale – reach for the skies as before and go up on your toes like you did last time and exhale and sweep your arms back to their original position by your side.

The important thing to remember is to use your breath to help you with the movements. One movement will be on the inhale while the next movement will be on the exhale. It is the energy of breath that helps you to achieve that wonderful feeling of pushing your body but you won't feel like you have pushed it too far because that's the wonderful thing about yoga. It isn't about punishment. It's about discipline and that's an entirely different thing.

Do this exercise five times and then relax. Go and stand in front of the mirror and I can almost guarantee that the person who looks back at you looks more confident than the original image. You will stand straighter, your waist and bodyline will look more flowing and you will feel sexier because of it.

There's something marvelous about yoga that you may not yet understand. When you muscles are stretched in this manner, it makes you a lot more versatile. Do you remember how certain sexual positions gave you cramp in the leg? Well, when they are exercised correctly, they won't give you this kind of problem anymore and your versatility and adaptability to different positions will enhance your sex life and make you much more adventurous.

I remember when I first started yoga, I had an appetite for the good things in life that was suddenly awaked in me. This included wanting to live my life to the fullest. My partner had to take up yoga to keep up with me! It's really good for the soul, but it's also good for self-image and if you feel better about the way that you look, you have fewer inhibitions. That automatically translates into being more sensual.

GRACE VERSUS TECHNIQUE

There are those who believe everything spiritual comes by grace. Yogis don't believe this. They believe that technique— the application of skilled effort and discipline—can alter the course of things and bring great well-being to our lives. However grace still plays a role. It is by grace that we are saved, the Bible teaches. Hindus would point to our **karma** from previous lives. Buddhists, who are in many ways the most direct descendants of the ancient yogis, would say it is by right knowledge and right action that we make spiritual progress. But whether by grace or because of inconsistent or faulty technique, we know that some days meditation comes easily and some days it doesn't come at all. Sometimes it really is best to take this simply as a matter of grace. Accept it, but don't stop meditating because of a bad day. Don't give up the practice of asana and **pranayama** just because some days it doesn't go well while other days, seemingly out of the blue when perhaps it is least expected, the bliss and the beauty, the joy and the understanding, are there almost without effort as though manna from heaven.

We should accept that too and continue our practice. The daily ebbs and flows, the highs and lows are best ignored and instead we should concentrate our effort on smoothing out our reaction to them and moving toward a time and place where all is bliss.

We should have a rational approach and a steady practice. We should have faith. It will come.

THE JOY OF THE EXPERIENCE

When you do yoga you will experience a heighten sense of consciousness. You will feel better. The world around you will be clearer, more brilliant. You will think better and life will be more enjoyable. In a way it's like being in love.

The changes will be both subtle and gross. On the one hand you will have to stop and notice the difference. You will have to practice awareness to see and feel the beauty. On the other hand you will suddenly become aware that everything today is very beautiful. You will exclaim, **I feel great and life is wonderful**. This won't happen all the time. Some days in the beginning it won't happen at all. But mostly it will. And as your practice deepens, so will your joy and so will the continuity of your experience. Life really is bliss and any deviation from that bliss (barring accident) is the result of error and ignorance. And even unfortunate accidents can be overcome and one's life made beautiful and full of joy through faith and practice.

Through a firm commitment and a gentle daily discipline, bad habits of mind and body melt away and inert flesh gives way to the effervescence of spirit.

SOME MISCONCEPTIONS

One of the major misconceptions about yoga is that it's an ascetic discipline. It's a discipline in the same sense that science is a discipline, but it's not austere, it's very pleasurable. In fact, pleasure is a constant goal of yoga, although the word "pleasure" is never used. Yogis are not in it for the pain. This misconception comes about because the yogi wants to actually transcend both pleasure and pain and reach bliss, "bliss" being a kind of superior pleasure not subject to the vagaries of the world (which the yogi knows he cannot control).

This is really the crux of the matter. What the yogi wants to do is to control his life so that he is not subject to the terrible ups and downs of triumph and disaster, of winning and losing—and to the extent that it is possible—the vagaries of pleasure and pain.

I remember a cartoon by Charles Schultz, the late artist who did "Peanuts," in which he has Lucy crying "I DON'T WANT any ups and downs! I want to go from up to UPs to...UPPER UPs!"

This is not exactly the way the yogi feels, but it illustrates the predicament so well expressed by Buddhism in the idea of **sukkha**, or the unsatisfactoriness of life.

Another misconception is that yoga is a uniquely Hindu phenomenon. Modern yoga is a synthesis of ideas and practices that come from India of course, but also from Tibet, from Taoist China, and from the far-flung provinces of Buddhism, including Japanese Zen Buddhism. The contemporary phenomenon that is yoga has been further influenced by Western ideas, principally the ideas of modern science. Thus an American yoga instructor would not say that the lotus posture destroys all disease or conquers death (as the classical authors of the **Hathapradipika** or the **Siva-Samhita** do) since that would be unscientific and perhaps misleading. Similarly, Western yogis do not practice, for example,

vahiskriti (washing the intestines) because this antiquated (and probably only symbolic) practice isn't necessary—or desirable!—in the modern world. The famous seated posture of yoga is the "lotus pose" not **padmasana** (its Sanskrit name). We say the "forward bend" not **paschimottanasana**. We clean our teeth with a toothbrush and toothpaste, not with catechu juice and clay (as prescribed in the **Gheranda-Samhita**).

Furthermore, Western instructors (not "gurus") typically limit themselves to teaching **hatha yoga**, leaving **raja** yoga to either the student himself or to a spiritual teacher (who could be Zen, Taoist, Christian, Hindu, Muslim or anything else).

While yoga's roots are in India, its full-flowering is world-wide.

WHAT YOGA IS NOT

Yoga is not something that can be gotten merely from books or film or from recordings or even ultimately from a guru.

Yoga is an experience. It is something learned with mind, body and soul. Although the outlines of yoga can be appreciated, and even its ultimate goal understood through verbal knowledge, the achievement of yoga can only be accomplished by doing yoga.

Yoga then is not the fakir who demonstrates his strength by sleeping on a bed of nails, nor is yoga the Hare Krishnas who used to come shaven-headed into the airports of prosperous countries to beg and intimidate passengers into giving them money (which they in turn gave to a controlling leader). Yoga is just the opposite. Instead of self-mutilation there is the practice of self-harmony. Instead of hustling for a fat and dictatorial "guru" (as sometimes happens in tantra) there is contentment with the self and no hustling at all.

THE APPROACH

It would be best (if it were possible) to come to yoga without preconceptions, to have tossed aside old ideas about what is important in life and to stand ready to begin anew, because to achieve yoga we will have to often embrace that which we previously shunned and to shun that which we previously held in highest esteem.

In this regard there is a symbol from the **Upanishads** of a tree stood upside down with its roots in the sky and its branches in the earth, signifying the diametric change in perception that comes about after one is firmly established in yoga.

A somewhat similar idea is from the Bible: "The meek shall inherit the earth." We have all heard this phrase many times, but have we ever stopped to ask what it really means? What is "meek" and what does it mean "to inherit?" What if I were to say to the CEO of a great international corporation that the meek shall inherit the earth?

The idea would probably annoy her. She would regard me as some kind of kook and/or Green fanatic out to deprive her of her corporate options. (Or maybe she would divine it as a great advertising idea!) If I reminded her that the quote is from the Bible she would probably come up with something like "the devil can quote scripture to his own purposes." At no time would she actually understand what I said nor would she have any idea of what was meant. She would only see that what I said was either in agreement with her world view or opposed to it; either as making her feel comfortable about her way of life or as reminding her that not everybody sees the world the way she does and that she might be wrong.

To achieve success in yoga we have to see as though for the first time, as a child experiences the world. We have to be willing intellectually and emotionally to be "born again."

But to be born again, one must first die to this world. One must allow the old delusive persona to expire so that the new might be born, like a chaparral forest burned to the ground so that an explosive spring of renewal might follow.

By the way, the meek are the modest, the non-violent, the peaceful. They are the wise who will survive after the merchants of war, exploitation, and intolerance are gone.

THE GOAL

The goal of yoga is **moksa**, freedom from pleasure and pain, from that tyrannical pair of opposites that control our lives. Put another way the goal of yoga is to merge with the Supreme Divine Consciousness, to become one with the Ineffable.

This is not exactly a modest undertaking! One might ask, do people actually achieve this? It's a good question and I hope this book provides something close to an answer. For moments, certainly, everyone has achieved **moksa**, everyone has been temporarily liberated. For some very rare persons such as Jesus or Buddha or Sri Ramakrishna or certain saints, the answer

73

is an unqualified yes. For weekend aspirants, the answer is probably not, at least not for a long time to come.

So what's the sense of trying?

The real beauty of yoga is that the benefits that one accrues along the way, even though one may come up far short of the goal, are themselves fabulous achievements: Good health, a serene and confident state of mind, a fuller understanding and appreciation of self, an acceptance of things one cannot control, a greater tolerance of others, an indifference toward evil, but compassion for those who suffer. (Evil, properly understood, is really just a delusion we can't help but believe.)

Contrary to some opinion, yoga is life-affirming. The practice of meditation (which is the core of yoga, as it is of all mystical experience) is not an escape from the world, but a way of ordering oneself into a greater harmony with the world. For the Hindu the goal is the cessation of the endless (and painful) cycle of birth, death and rebirth. For the yogi the expression is more direct. It is pure bliss itself, a heaven on earth.

The first goal, then, is physical health. Toward that end, we practice asana and **pranayama**, we live in harmony with our fellow human beings, we meditate. For the experienced aspirant the goal is **samadhi**, the achievement of the super conscious state that is beyond the power of words to describe. (Although we rationalists might just call it "trance," as it is sometimes translated, and leave it at that.) For the saint it is union with the Supreme Divine Consciousness.

How do we know that Sri Ramakrishna and Jesus, for example, actually achieved this union with God?

We know nothing of course except our own experience, but we can gain trust from the pure veracity of their words. Jesus said, "Seek ye the Kingdom of Heaven within." How did he know that the

Kingdom of Heaven was within? He knew because he himself had experienced the Kingdom first hand.

We further have the reports of their disciples to the truth of their experiences. Ramakrishna went into trances of ecstasy sometimes for months on end. His disciples were there with him to share his experience and to experience the wonder (second hand at least). When he spoke during these periods what he said was so charged with truth and the terrific desire to lead others to where he had been that one could hardly doubt that he spoke from personal experience. He was asked how to see God and he said you must cry to him with a yearning heart, and you will see him.

Later he told a story about a guru and his disciple. The disciple too wanted to see God, so the guru took him down to the river and held his head underwater a long time. When he let him up, the guru asked how he felt. The student said, "'Oh, I thought I should die; I was panting for breath!' The teacher said, 'When you feel like that for God, then you will know you haven't long to wait for His vision.'"

But I think the reader should be skeptical. Trust only your own experience and use the experience of others only as a guide. But remember the great psychological truth in the adage, "None are so blind as those who will not see."

IS YOGA A RELIGION?

Surprisingly this is a controversial question—at least in the United States. Most popular yoga books in English are at pains to say that yoga is not a religion and point out that one can practice yoga and still be a Christian or a Buddhist—or an atheist—and it will make no difference. But maybe it would be wiser to see yoga not as a religion per se but as something that aids one in his religious practice. To quote Gopi Krishna from his book, **The Secret of Yoga**, p. 2:

Properly speaking, yoga is an adjunct to religion and has always been treated as such in India.... Yoga is not something different or divorced from religion. It is the experimental part of it....

He adds:

Divested of the superstition and myth that surround all religions, Yoga contains absolutely nothing that can be abhorrent to any faith or creed. On the other hand, it uses most of the methods advocated by the founders of great religions, mystics, and sages as a means to God-consciousness and to render the body as a fit vehicle for spiritual illumination.

WHAT YOGA IS

Yoga is a spiritual practice, an ancient tradition, a science, a religion, a way of life. It is all of these things. Its literature is vast, its lineage ancient, its scope all-encompassing, taking as it does into consideration every aspect of a person's life.

The word yoga itself means "to bind" or "to attach" or "yoke," as to yoke oxen. In a deeper sense it means to yoke the individual soul to God.

It has been called "a poise of the soul" (Mahadev Desai) or "the establishment of perfect harmony between the everyday self and its spiritual source" (Paul Brunton, in Wood's **Practical Yoga**, p. 10).

Patanjali himself defined yoga tersely as "the control of the ideas of the mind."

Dr. Ramurti S. Mishra says that man is "hypnotized by his body" (I like that phrasing) and calls yoga "the process of dehypnotism." He adds that "submission of lower desire to higher desire is called yoga."

In the **Bhagavad Gita** yoga is described as "a deliverance from contact with pain and sorrow."

On a more practical level, the **hatha yoga** teacher Indra Devi called yoga "a method, a system of physical, mental and spiritual development" (**Yoga for Americans**, p. xxii).

Georg Feuerstein in the Preface to **The Shambhala Encyclopedia of Yoga** identifies yoga as "an immensely rich and highly complex spiritual tradition...."

In his **Yoga: Immortality and Freedom**, Mircea Eliade says, "The means of attaining to Being, the effectual techniques for gaining liberation. This...constitutes Yoga properly speaking."

Secularly speaking, then, one might say that yoga is a growing body of knowledge and practice that teaches people to live in harmony with themselves and their environment. Spiritually speaking, some yogis say (as Sachindra Kumar Majumdar did in his **Introduction to Yoga**, p. 20) that "Yoga is the religion of mankind." But this would be going too far.

Yoga is also one of the six orthodox philosophies of Hinduism.

A WAY OF LIFE

As you can surmise, every book on yoga attempts to define what yoga is. All these attempts are fine, but what they usually fail to tell the reader is that to understand what yoga is you have to practice yoga, and I don't mean merely the postures. A definition won't tell you. Reading a book, any book, including this one, won't tell you. You have to live yoga to appreciate what yoga is.

In the beginning of course words help. Yoga is not an exotic herb. That's good to know. Yoga is not an ice cream sundae. Yoga is a practice, of course, as I said above, but more than that yoga is a way of life.

A way of life. These are small words, but their intent is to cover everything. All of life, every experience, every stage, everything we do or say, every experience we have, correctly understood, is covered in yoga.

Sound all-inclusive? That was the intent of the ancient yogis. The science, art and practice of yoga is intended to guide us through everything that life can throw at us, from birth to death. Yoga is a way to meet what life has to offer, yoga is a way of viewing what happens to us, yoga is a theory about what happens to us, yoga is a guide on how to live in this world and how to die.

However words do not suffice. It is only through direct experience that we may know what yoga is.

So let us begin.

Chapter 8: Embarking On Your Yoga Weight Loss Program

Stress, as we have already determined, is an inescapable part of our lives. We have also determined that it is a cause for accumulation of fat. You are probably going to the gym every morning before starting on your stressful day. You might even have had a healthy breakfast and are planning to eat healthy for the rest of the day. Research has revealed that even if you eat healthy and exercise, chronic stress can prevent you from losing weight...and even cause you to gain pounds.

Everyone's body responds in the same way. Each time you experience stress, your brain instructs your cells to release the hormones we discussed about earlier. You get a burst of adrenaline which taps stored energy. This is accompanied by a surge of cortisol, which directs your body to replenish that energy even though you haven't actually used that many calories. This is because our bodies were created to respond and react to threats like wild animal attacks, etc. When the adrenaline is released, our bodies are geared to run.

Stress, while similarly prompting the release of adrenaline, obviously doesn't cause you to run, because the attack you are under is of a different kind than, say, a cheetah attack. Therefore, when the cortisol surge takes place, you haven't burned any calories by running, but you are hungry, since the cortisol is telling your body to replenish the energy which your stressful encounter might have caused you to use. Had you been a prehistoric caveman or cavewoman running from predators, you would have spent energy by release of adrenalin and the cortisol would have informed you to eat, because you have been through a stressful – fight or flight - situation. Imagine this – your body is continuing to pump out cortisol as long as you are under stress.

Thus, you find yourself "stress eating", and the destructive part about this cycle is that you seldom reach for healthy food when you are in this state, but instead crave sweet, salty and high fat foods because they stimulate your brain to release 'pleasure chemicals' that reduce tension. What adds further negativity to this situation is that when the 'pleasure chemicals' are released, you feel calm and soothed, so every time another stress attack hits you, you're reaching for chocolate and ice cream. Believe me, it's not just a cycle but a vicious cycle, because cortisol also encourages your body to store fat, especially visceral fat which is very dangerous, as it surrounds vital organs and releases fatty acids into your blood, raising cholesterol and insulin levels and causing heart disease and diabetes, amongst other life threatening diseases.

You have good news here! You can actually reverse this situation if you turn to Yoga.

You need to achieve balance of body, mind and soul

When you begin the study or practice of Yoga, you will learn that our bodies are divided into seven 'Chakras' or focus points of energy. If these are thrown out of sync it results in a lot of stress, anger, irritation, unbalanced behavior like overeating, etc. It is therefore of the utmost importance to keep our chakras balanced. Balanced chakras enable energy to flow freely from one point of our body to the other. Blocked chakras inhibit the flow of energy and gets in the way of our equilibrium. When our equilibrium is upset, our bodies don't process our food efficiently and our metabolism is not working at peak. The result is weight gain. Regular practitioners of Yoga and Yogic Meditation have lean bodies and alert, bright eyes. This is because their chakras are always in a state of balance— the kind of balance that promotes weight loss without indulging in stress inducing workouts.

Thoroughly understand the Seven Chakras

Sahasrara Chakra: This Chakra is at the top of the head and relates to Understanding and Will.

Ajna Chakra: This is directly behind the centre of the forehead, in the position of the 'third eye'. It relates to Intuition.

Visuddha Chakra: This is in the throat area and is connected to Power

Anahata Chakra: This is situated at the center of the chest and has to do with relationships, love, forgiveness, compassion, self-control and self-acceptance.

Manipura Chakra: This Chakra is situated above the navel in the stomach area. It is connected with wisdom, balance of intellect, self-confidence, self-control and humor.

Svadishthana Chakra: This is located in the lower abdomen, below the navel. It relates to order.

Muladhara Chakra: This is located at the base of the spine or coccyx. It has to do with life and survival.

Alignment of the Chakras leads to harmony and wellbeing, but when the Chakras are out of balance a variety of physical, mental and emotional imbalances impact the system. The imbalance of the Chakras manifests itself in depression, fatigue, eating disorders, alcohol abuse, asthma, allergies, digestive disorders, thyroid problems, hormonal imbalances, mood swings, etc.

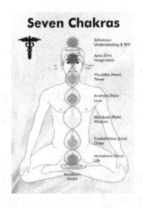

88

Yoga practices deliver innumerable health benefits but it's not a substitute of medicine. It is a natural and zero side effect approach towards healthy living. Regular yoga practices restore physical and mental health. Yoga enhances the quality of life by reinstalling vigor. Yoga improves overall well-being by promoting, weight loss, glowing beautiful skin, good health, flexible body and peaceful mind. It minimizes the symptoms of discomfort and illness and combats negative emotions. Yoga operates in a four–way approach that includes:

Physical. Yoga strengthens and heals the skeletal, digestive, muscular, nervous, cardio-vascular, lymphatic, excretory and endocrine system by stretching and relaxing. The yoga exercises deliver lean, strong, long and confident body.

Mental. The deep breaths renovates the mind to its crude and natural form by restoring peace, concentration and alertness. Yoga nurtures the mind and keeps it sharp, focused and calm. Yoga is the practice of quieting the mind-Patanjali.

Psychological. Yoga illuminates our tendencies and behaviour. It nourishes freedom of choice. Regular and religious yoga practices inspire us to ameliorate and revamp our lives by fostering devotion, courage and ingenuity.

Spiritual. The beautiful and wondrous experience of meditation (integral part of yoga), revitalizes our inner peace with compassion, goodwill and kindness. This relaxed state of mind further boast affection, generosity and humanity.

Ymber Delecto said that 'Yoga is invigoration in relaxation, freedom in routine, confidence through self-control, energy within and energy without. Thus, to recognize the potential and power of yoga, it is critical to understand its multiple benefits. Some of them are listed below:

Yoga and Diabetes-Stress, unhealthy and un-appropriate food habits and lack of physical exercise give birth to Diabetes. This disorder marked by increase in the level of glucagon (hormone of the pancreas that enhances sugar levels in blood). The fast paced life aggravates the symptoms of Diabetes. However, by incorporating yogic practices that includes pranayam, meditation and yoga in the daily and regular regime is a step towards better mental, physical and mental health. Regularity and consistency can bring sterling and splendid results. Some of the effective pranayam and asana for Diabetes cure and treatment are:

Kapal Bhati Pranayam (Skull shining breathing technique)

Dharunasana (Upward wheel pose)

Chakrasana (Wheel pose)

Paschimottanaasana (seated forward bend)

Shavasana (corpse pose)

Yoga and Digestion. The sole pillar of a healthy and salubrious lifestyle is a proper and good digestive system. A healthy and robust digestive system alleviates physical ailments such as stomach ache, constipation, acnes, ulcers, bloating and pimples. A faulty digestive system is an outcome of unhealthy food habits, hectic lifestyle and over-eating. It is important to maintain positivity and patience. Regular practice of yoga is proven to improve digestion. A few yoga exercise essential for healthy digestive system are:

Ustrasana (Camel pose)

Naukasana (Boat pose)

Setu Bandhasana (Bridge pose)

Padmasana (Lotus pose)

Pavanakutasana (Wind Relieving Pose)

Yoga and Fertility. Yoga offers multi-fold benefits on regular practice. Excessive strenuous work load, tight jam-packed schedules, thirst for growth appraisals and mind-numbing long work hours have taken a toll of our beautiful lives. High and elevated levels of stress hamper the body's fertility in both men and women. The chances of conception (baby) significantly contracts due to depression, stress, anxiety and guilt. Practicing yoga enhances conception chances as it tones and strengthens our mind, body and soul. Yoga fosters calm mind and hospitable body for the baby. Certain yoga exercise or postures would trigger towards the path of parenthood by improving the fertility level are:

Nadi Shodhan Prayanam (Alternate Nostril Breathing)

Hastapadasana(standing forward bend)

Bhramari Pranayam (bee breath)

Yoga Nidra (Yogic sleep)

Badkakonasana(butterfly pose)

Yoga and Blood Pressure. Yoga lowers the blood pressure as it's co-related with peace of mind and relaxation. It is superior to other forms of physical activities and exercise for curing high blood pressure as it has positive effect on anxiety and mood. The temporary rise in blood pressure occurs due to over-exposure to anger, stress, mental tension and excessive thinking. A complete and comprehensive program of Yoga asana and pranayamas is effective to combat high blood pressure naturally. Here are few:

Sukhasan (Easy or pleasant pose)

Ardh-Halasan (Half-plough pose)

Shishu Asana (Child Pose)

Vajrasan (Kneeling or Diamond Pose)

Pawankuktasana (circular movements)

Yoga and Arthritis. Ageing aggregates the symptoms of arthritis and joint pain. Lack of adequate exercise, weak bone structure and deficiency of essential and vital nutrients worsen the condition. Certain medicines though alleviate the pain but the ancient Indian technique of Yoga eliminates the pain permanently. Yoga calms the stressed mind, tones the disputed body and heals the pain. As it triggers emotional, mental wellbeing by fostering ameliorating the joint health. Yoga has a significant positive impact in the quality of our lives. Arthritis patients enjoy yoga over other physical and traditional forms of exercises. It is a supreme natural method to successfully beating stiffness, discomfort and joint pain. This set of asanas, is proven to beat arthritis effectively.

Veerbhadrasana (Warrior Pose)

Trikonasana (Triangle pose)

Ustrasana (Camel Pose)

Dhanusasana (Bow Pose)

Yoga and Irritable Bowel Syndrome. Irritable Bowel Syndrome is described as a physical disorder characterized by prolonged discomfort, abdominal pain, diarrhea, bloating, constipation and abnormal bowel movements. It is common in both men, women and children but women are more susceptible. This gastro-intestinal tract disorder disturbs the quality of life and often, leads to mental and emotional stress. Yoga helps to relive this ailment as this ancient technique works at psychical and psychological level. Some yoga exercises which prove beneficial for Irritable Bowel Syndrome are:

Marjariasana (Cat pose)

Bhujangasana (Cobra pose)

Ardha Matsyendrasana (Sitting Half-Spinal Twist)

Adho Mukha Shvasasana (Downward Facing Dog Pose)

Dhanursana (Bow Pose)

Yoga and Sleep. Yoga is an anxiety alleviating and relaxation tool and restores the body to its optimum condition. Yoga is known and proven to cure abnormal sleeping habits and insomnia. It significantly unwinds stress levels. Sleep deprivation is a critical source of concern and stress amongst the people as stress and sleep are vicious cycle. Yoga lowers the stress levels, relives tension and calms the mind as it's a natural, soothing sleep inducing remedy. It combats insomnia and restlessness. Some important sleep inducing Yoga exercises are:

Sukhasana (Easy forward bend)

Uttanasana (Standing forward bend)

Balasana (Child Pose)

Viparita Karani (Legs up the wall pose)

Savasana (Corpse pose)

Yoga for Eyes. Yoga helps to overcome eye-related problems by improving and enhancing the functioning of eyes. It is helpful in short sightedness (Myopia), Long sightedness (Hypermetropia), glaucoma, cataract and other bacterial infection diseases. Certain eye related disorders occur due to the malfunctioning and disturbance of ocular muscles, caused by emotional and mental tensions. Yoga techniques restrict eye related disorder and defects. Some therapeutic yoga techniques that enhance eye functioning are:

Blinking

Palming

Near and Distant Viewing

Rotational Viewing

Preliminary nose tip gazing

Yoga for Hair Loss. Hair condition and health is the barometer of our own health. Main reasons for hair loss are ageing, hormonal imbalance, genetics, stress, unhealthy lifestyle, medication and over-exposure to hair care products. Yoga practices restrict hair loss, stimulates healthy scalp and motivates hair re-growth. Beautiful hair makes you look attractive and improves your overall personality .Yoga enhances blood circulation to the scalp and thus, promotes hair growth. Yoga also restores our crowing beauty (hair) by strengthening the existing hair in our scalp. Some of the useful yoga exercises are:

Balayam Yoga (Rubbing Nails)

Uttanasana (Stand forward bend pose)

Sasangasana (Rabbit Pose)

Adho Mukha Svanasana (Downward Dog Pose)

Matsyanasana (Fish pose)

Yoga and Heart. Heart diseases are an outcome of very little or no exercise, poor stress management, consumption of fatty food and sedentary lifestyle. Yoga techniques are beneficial for retarding chronic coronary artery diseases if effectively incorporated with dietary modification, stress management coupled with lifestyle reforms. Yoga improves the overall blood circulation while pranayam restores better and effective breathing. The meditation involved with yoga helps in rejuvenation and relaxation of our mind. Aa yoga postures affect our respiratory system, therefore t has a positive impact on our heart. A few yoga exercises that affect our heart positively are:

Tadasana (Mountain pose)

Utthita Hastapadasana (Extended hands and feet pose)

Vrikshasana (Tree pose)

Veerabhadrasana (Warrior Pose)

Bhujangasana (Cobra Pose)

Yoga for Migraine. Yoga enhances our resistance towards the unbearable pain of migraine. This neurological disorder is characterized by recurring unbearable headaches of moderate and high intensity. Migraine triggers light and sound sensitivity in the patient. The pain can last for two hours or even two or more days. Migraine is more common than diabetes, asthma and epilepsy. Yoga can cure this neurological disorder and even, prevent migraine attacks. As majority of the headaches are tension related, Yoga works by relieving and uprooting the stress and tension. Yoga improves the blood circulation and hence, supplies more oxygen to the brain.

Shishuasana (Child Pose)

Hastapadasana (Standing forward bend)

Marjariasana (Cat stretch)

Setu Bandhasana (Bridge pose)

Padmasana (Lotus pose)

Yoga for Asthma. Yoga is natural asthma relief. Patients of asthma suffer from bronchocontriction (exercise induced).Therefore, Yoga is gaining immense popularity, as it is a blend of slow pace exercise, gentle stretches and an effective stress relieving technique. Yoga improves the lung function and alleviates asthma symptoms. Yoga is all about physical, mental and spiritual relaxation. It is believed in Yoga philosophy that a calm mind induces regular breathing and hence, fosters a relaxed body. Therefore, the breathing exercise of Yoga helps to deal with Bronchitis and Asthma. Yoga is a good therapy for respiratory ailment and problems. As yoga involves Pranayama (art of breath control) and Asanas (body postures), it benefits the people with respiratory disorders and enhances overall well-being. A few yoga exercises beneficial for Asthma patients are:

Nadi Shodhan pranayam (Alternate nostril breathing technique)

Kapal Bhati Pranayam (Skull shining breathing technique)

Pavanmuktasana (Wind Relieving pose)

Adho Mukha Svanasana (Downward facing dog pose)

Bhujangasana (Cobra Pose)

Yoga for Thyroid. Thyroid disease has become a widespread disorder after, diabetes and hypertension. Its prevalence rate in higher in women than in men .The sole cause of thyroid disorders are stressful and sedentary lifestyle. Yoga and meditation are an excellent remedy to cope up with the thyroid disorder. Regular yoga practices uproot stress levels and thus, promote a happy and smooth life. There are two main types of thyroid disorder namely Hypothyroidism (underactive thyroid) and Hyperthyroidism (over-active thyroid).Pranayamas (breathing techniques) such as Nadi Shodhan Pranayama (alternate nostril breathing technique), Kapal Bhati Pranayama (skull shining breathing technique) Ujjayi and Bhastrika help in reducing the symptoms of thyroid. Yoga Nidra is beneficial fop hypothyroidism and hyperthyroidism as it works by relaxing and calming down the mind. Some Yoga Postures effective for thyroid disorders are:

☐ Hypothyroidism

Sarvangasana (Shoulder Stand)

Halasana (Plow Pose)

Surya Namaskar (Fast-paced Sun Salutation)

Janu Shirasasana (One-legged Forward Bend)

Marjarisasana (Cat Stretch)

☐ Hyperthyroidism

Shavasana (Corpse pose)

Shishu Asana (Child Pose)

Surya Namaskar (Slow paced Sun salutation)

Marjariasana (Cat stretch)

Setubandhsana (Bridge Pose)

Yoga and Smoking. All of us know smoking is injurious to our health as the smoke inhaled shelters 4000 chemicals. Most of these chemicals are carcinogenic (cancer causing). According, to the statistic of WHO (World Health Organization). Tobacco is the sole reason of 6 million deaths, every year. Despite the awareness of the adverse effects of smoking tobacco, smokers find it hard to quit this bad habit. The critical reason for tobacco addiction is its ability to relax the mind and provide temporary peace from the stress. However, Yoga is an excellent therapy to aid your way to non-addiction and de-stressing. Yoga is a prominent wellness program, designed to enrich our health. You should blow away the smoke by incorporating certain pranayamas and yoga postures listed below for your way to quit smoking:

Sarvangasana (Shoulder stand)

Bhujanagasana (Cobra pose)

Nadi Shodhan Pranayama (Alternate nostril breathing technique)

Kapal Bhati Pranayama (Skull Shining Breathing Technique)

Setu Bandhasana (Bridge Pose)

Yoga and Mind. Yoga and meditation help us to explore the peace, within us. It restores our serenity, peace and natural beauty. It has high potential to calm, a disturbed mind. Yoga is an ancient secret of being energetic and fresh, as it keeps the mind, body and soul recharged and refreshed, even during hectic schedules. Yoga yields significant positive results to reinforce intuition. It strengthens the relationship with parents, spouse, friends and loved ones. It prepares the mind to deal with sensitive and tough relationship issues by promoting contentment, happiness and relaxation. Yoga strengthens bonds and helps to build strong connections. Yoga enriches our awareness as it works by releasing the stress. Yoga is truly a doubt-repeller, mind soother and most importantly, a creativity booster machine. Some incredible benefits of asanas and pranayamas for our mind are:

Boosts self esteem

Magnifies alertness and peace

Strengthens the energy levels and enthusiasm

Escalates confidence

Develops focus

Promotes good memory

Enhances the ability to cope with stress and addiction

Augments decision making ability

Stimulates concentration

Yoga for Beauty. Yoga aids to beautify the skin. Yoga stimulates blood circulation and hence, is perfect solution for beautiful face, body and mind. Yoga can help you flaunt radiating, flawless and healthy skin that mesmerizes and catches attention. It is free from harmful chemicals and expensive beauty treatments as its 100% natural and side-effect free remedy. Certain harmful lifestyle practices like alcohol, smoking, unhealthy food habits and drug addiction cause premature ageing and wrinkles. Hormonal imbalances and improper digestion give rise to acne. However, with yoga practices, blood circulation enhances to our face and head. Thus, it supplies more oxygen to our cells and helps us achieve glowing and clean skin. Certain paranayamas provide a cooling and soothing effect in summers and helps to combat oily skin and hence, retains the glow. Yoga is beneficial as it's facilitates emotional and physical cleansing. Some popular postures of yoga help to detox the body naturally by its forceful and strong exhalation process and thus promotes natural glow. Meditation, involved in Yoga, fosters the body to radiate from within and thus, brings charm in our face. Religious practices of Yoga tighten the facial muscles and reduces sagging. Some yoga exercise effective for an enchanting and attractive beauty are:

Anulom Vilom Pranayama (Alternate Nostril Breathing)

Kapal Bhati Pranayama (Skull Shining Breathing Technique)

Surya Namaskar(Sun Salutation)

Bhujanagasana(Cobra Pose)

Trikonasana (Triangle Pose)

CHAPTER 10: SETTING THE PACE– THE SUN SALUTATION AND WARM UP POSES

The Sun Salutation is a kind of warm up exercise that is consist of 12 positions. These positions prepare the body for the succeeding yoga session. Each position brings about different vertebral movement to the spine and is pitched to the inhalation and exhalation thereby infusing balance and harmony. The positions are easy to follow. Make six sequences at the beginning of each yoga session and tune the sequence to your breath.

The Prayer Pose

Stand up straight with both feet together. Inhale and then exhale as you bring your palms in a prayer-like position at chest level.

The Arch Back

Still in a standing position, arch your back with your hips coming forward, and then slowly stretch your arms up over your head aligning your ears. Stretch as far as your body can.

Bend Over

This is the third sun salutation position and you must extend your body and bend down reaching your toes whilst exhaling. Your hips must be kept up high as you bend and your forehead tucked in between your legs. And then, bring your both hands touching the floor and place them on the sides of your feet.

Leg Back

Inhale as you stretch your right leg at the back and then bend your left knee. Lift your head up while your hands must be positioned either at the side of your foot. Throughout the pose, your hands must be placed that way.

Push-up pose

This kind of yoga pose strengthens the arms, back and core, as well as the abdominals. Start by taking on the push up position with your left foot back next to your right foot. Keep the spine and elbows straight and do not let the hips and head drop. Retain your breath as you do the pose.

Lower your upper body to the floor

Still taking on the push-up position, exhale as you lower both knees to the floor while the hips must be completely off the ground. Keep your chest straight. If you are a beginner, you may try lowering down your chin instead of your forehead.

Arch the chest

With your chest against the floor, slowly slide your body up and forward. The chest must be arched forward and the head tilt at the back. Your elbows must be slightly bent.

The Inverted V

This is the 8th position in the sun salutation. Begin by coming into an inverted V pose by raising your hips, both knees straight and your hands extended forward. As you assume the position, remember to do it without rocking the body.

Lunge forward

Take a deep breath as you take on the lunge position and bring your right foot forward in between your hands. Drop your left knee with the front of your foot on the floor. Raise your head and look up the ceiling.

Forehead to knees

Breathe out as you bring your left foot forward next to your right foot with the tips of your fingers forming a straight line. Slowly raise your hips whilst keeping the hands in the same position. Remember to keep your legs straight as you do the pose. But if you are a beginner, you may slightly bend your knees, but the hips must remain up all throughout. Tuck your head in between your knees and bring it down for as low as you can manage.

Stretch back

Begin in a standing position and inhale as you come into a full stretch, but this time, arching your back into a full curve and stretching your arms above your head. Your arms must be parallel to the ears, arch chest forward, knees straight and feet together.

Return to starting position

This is the final sun salutation exercise. Exhale as you straighten up your body, lower your hands to the side, and prepare for another sun salutation sequence.

CHAPTER 11: YOGA POSES FOR WEIGHT LOSS

1) Bridge Pose (Sethu Bandh Asana)

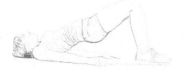

Fig. 1.1 Bridge Pose

Instructions to practice this yoga pose :-

Follow the below instructions step by step.

Step-1: First of all lie on your back.

Step-2: Fold your knees and keep your feet hip distance apart on the floor, It should be 10-12 inches from your pelvis, with knees and ankles in a straight line.

Step-3: **Now** keep your arms beside your body, palms facing down.

Step-4: Inhale and lift your inner back, middle back and upper back off the floor slowly. Now gently roll in the shoulders; touch the chest to the chin without bringing the chin down, supporting your weight with your shoulders, arms and feet. Feel your bottom firm up in this pose. Both the thighs should be parallel to each other and to the floor.

Step-5: As variation you could interlace the fingers and push the hands on the floor to lift the torso a little more up, or you could support your back with your palms.

Step-6: Always keep breathing easy.

Step-7: You could hold the posture for 1 or 2 minutes and then release with exhale.

Precautions:

1. Pregnant women should practice carefully under the doctor's guidance and should not practice with full force during pregnancy.

2. Your legs and feet should be parallel.

3. If you are having injuries to the neck, shoulder or spine then you should not practice this pose.

Other Important Benefits:

1. This yoga pose strengthens the back muscles and relieves the tired back instantaneously.

2. It gives good stretch to the neck, spine and chest.

3. It also helps digestion process of your body.

2) Frog Pose (Bhek-asana)

Frog pose is a great pose if you want to shed pounds from your hips and buttocks. It is a simple yet very effective posture to stretch and open your hips, groin and the inside of your thighs.

Instructions to perform this pose:-

Step-1: **First of all** lie on your belly and place both your forearms on the floor parallel to the mat.

Step-2: After this bend both your knees and point your toes towards the ceiling.

Step-3: Now stretch your arms behind and try to grab both your feet with your hands.

Step-4: Start inhaling slowly and lift your chest as high as you can, squeezing your shoulders towards one another. The higher you lift your chest, the easier it will be for you to hold your feet.

Step-5: You should maintain this position for 10-15 seconds and then release your body to the ground and relax.

Precautions:

1. You should avoid doing this pose if you have had a recent injury to your knees, hips and legs.

2. You should do this pose gradually because it is helpful in lower back flexibility.

Other Benefits:

1. This pose also opens up the hip joints of your body.

2. It is the best pose for strength of your lower back.

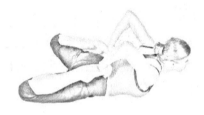

Fig-1.2 Frog Pose

3) Bow Pose (Dhanurasana)

Instructions to perform this pose:

Step-1: First step is to lie on your stomach with your feet hip-width apart and your arms by the side of your body.

Step-2: Now fold your knees and hold your ankles.

Step-3: Inhale and lift your chest off the ground and pull your legs up and back.

Step-4: Now look ahead. Curve of your lips should match to curve of your body.

Step-5: Maintain this pose while paying attention to your breath. Your body is now taut as a bow.

Step-6: Keep taking long deep breaths as you relax in this pose. But do not overdo the stretch.

Step-7: You should maintain this pose for 15-20 seconds after that while exhaling gently bring your legs and chest to the ground . Now release the ankles and relax.

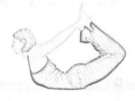

Fig 1.3 Bow Pose

Precautions:

1. You should not practice this pose if you have high or low blood pressure, hernia, any neck injury, pain in the lower back.

2. Ladies should avoid practicing this pose during pregnancy.

3. If you have migraine or any lower back injury you must not practice this pose.

Other benefits:

1. This pose is very helpful for greater flexibility to the back.

2. Bow pose also stimulates the reproductive organs and relieves menstrual discomfort. and constipation.

3. Those who are suffering from renal(kidney) disorders should practice this pose and find the great help.

4) Cobra Pose (Bhujangasana)

Instructions to perform this pose:

Step-1: First step is to lie down on the stomach. Keep your legs together by making a gap of 1-2 feet between the legs if somebody has backache.

Step-2: Now put your palms besides shoulder and your head should rest on the ground.

Step-3: While inhaling raise your head up as high as you can to your navel region and try to see the roof.

Step-4: Now maintain the position for 10-60 seconds with steadily taking breath in and out.

Step-5: After this come the original position slowly and relax.

Step-6: Repeat the process for 3 to 5 times.

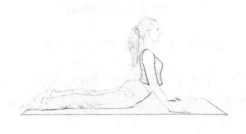

Fig.1.4 Cobra Pose

Precautions:

1. Pregnant women should not perform this pose.

2. If you have abdominal injuries then avoid doing this pose.

3. The person who is suffering from hernia, intestinal tuberculosis, hypothyroidism and peptic ulcers shouldn't practice this pose.

Other benefits:

1. This pose ensures the better health by facilitating the effective coordination between the brain and rest of your body parts.

2. This pose also helps in improving the efficiency of kidney by removing the stagnated blood.

5) Chair Pose (Utkatasana)

Instructions to perform this pose:

Step-1: First of all stand with your feet together, with your big toes touching. To make this step easy beginners can stand with their feet hip-distance apart.

Step-2: While Inhaling raise your arms above your head, it should be perpendicular to the floor.

Step-3: Now breathe out as you bend your knees, bring your thighs as parallel to the floor as they can get. Your knees will project out slightly over your feet and your torso will form approximately a right angle over your thighs.

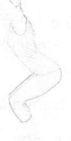

Fig. 1.5 Chair Pose

Step-4: Now draw your shoulder blades into your upper back ribs as you reach your elbows back towards your ears. Do not puff your ribcage forward. Draw your tailbone down to the floor, and keep your lower back long.

Step-6: While bring your hips down even lower lift through your heart. There should be a slight bend in your upper back.

Step-7: Now shift your weight into your heels.

Step-8: Keep your breath smooth, even, and deep. Back off a bit in the pose if breathe has become shallow or strained.

Step-9: While spreading your shoulder blades apart spin your fingers toward each other so your palms face each other. Now rotate your arms outward through your thumbs.

Step-10: Now gaze directly forward. Tilt your head slightly and gaze at a point between your hands for a deeper pose.

Step-11: You should hold this pose for one minute. Then, breathe in as you straighten your legs, lifting through your arms. Breathe out and come back to initial state.

Beginner's Tip:

1. You can practice it near a wall to help you remain in the pose. You can stand with your back towards the wall and a few inches away from it.

2. You should maintain an appropriate distance so that when you come into position, your tailbone touches the wall and is supported by it.

Precautions:

1. Those suffering from low pressure, insomnia, and headaches must avoid this pose.

2. If you are having any shoulder injury, you should make sure to practice this pose with care.

3. If you cannot raise your arms over your head without experiencing pain then move only within the areas where you don't feel the pain.

Other benefits:

1. This pose exercises the spine, chest and hip muscles.

2. Practice of this pose helps in strengthen the torso and lower back.

3. This pose tones the thigh, leg, ankle and knee muscles.

6) Warrior Pose I (Virbhadrasana)

Instructions to perform this pose:

Step-1: First of all stand straight with your legs wide apart by a distance of at least 3-4 feet.

Step-2: Now turn your right foot out by 90 degrees and left foot in by about 15 degrees.You right foot should be aligned to the center of the left foot.

Step-3: Now lift both of your arms sideways to shoulder height with your palms facing upwards. Your arms should be parallel to the ground.

Step-4: While exhaling bend your right knee. Your right knee and right ankle should form a straight line and ensure that your knee does not overshoot the ankle.

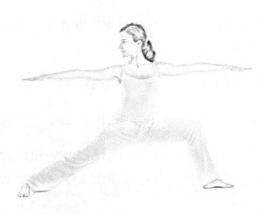

Fig. 1.6 Warrior Pose

Step-5: Turn your head and look to your right.

Step-6: As you settle down in the yoga posture stretch your arms further.

Step-7: Now make a gentle effort to push your pelvis down. Maintain the yoga posture with the determination of a warrior. Smile like a happy smiling warrior. Keep breathing smoothly as you go down.

Step-8: While inhaling come up and while exhaling bring your hands down from the sides.

Step-9: Perform the same steps for the left side (turn your left foot out by 90 degrees and turn the right foot in by about 15 degrees).

Precautions:

1. If you are suffering from diarrhoea then avoid practice of this pose.

2. If you have experienced spinal disorders recently or just recovered from a chronic

illness then practice only after consulting your doctor.

Other Benefits:

1. This pose is beneficial for those with deskbound jobs.

2. This yoga posture is extremely beneficial in case of frozen shoulders.

7) Boat Pose (Naukasana)

Instructions to perform this pose:

Step-1: First step is to lie on your back with your feet together and arms beside your body.

Step-2: Now take a deep breath in and as you breathe out lift your chest and feet off the ground and stretch your arms towards your feet.

Step-3: Your eyes, fingers and toes should be in a line.

Step-4: You will feel the tension in your navel area as the abdominal muscles contract.

Step-5: Maintain this pose and keep the breath deep and even.

Step-6: Now come back to the ground while exhaling and then relax.

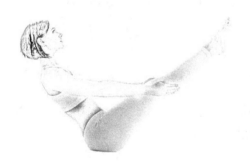

Fig.1.7 Boat Pose

Precautions:

1. If you are suffering from asthma or heart diseases then avoid this poise.

2. Pregnant woman should avoid this pose and during the first 2 days of the menstrual cycle.

Other benefits:

1. This pose strengthens the abdominal muscles and your back.

2. This pose also tones the leg and arm muscles.

3. Best yoga posture for people with hernia.

8) Mountain Pose (Tadasana)

Instructions to perform this pose:

Step-1: First stand straight on a mat.

Step-2: Now put your hands up and stretch as much as you can. You should try to keep your hands straight.

Step-3: Maintain this pose few seconds.

Step-4: After this put your hands down and come back to initial state. Relax.

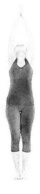

Fig. 1.8 Mountain Pose

Other benefits:

1. This is the most recommended practice for increasing height of body.

9) Half-Moon Pose (Ardha chandraasana)

Instructions to perform this pose:

Step-1: First step is to stand with your feet together.

Step-2: Now raise your hands above your head and clasp palm together. Try to extend the stretch by trying to reach ceiling.

Step-3: While exhaling slowly bend sideways from your hips and keep your hands together. Do not bend forward and keep your elbows straight. You should feel a stretch from your fingertips to your thighs.

Step-4: Now inhale and come back to the standing position.

Step-5: Repeat this pose for other side.

Step-6: Relax.

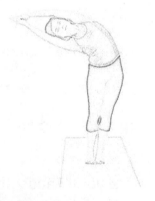

Fig. 1.9 Half-Moon Pose

Precautions:

1. If you have digestive disorders, a spine injury or high blood pressure then avoid doing this pose.

Other benefits:

1. This pose is great for your inner and upper thigh.

2. This pose helps burn off unsightly love handles and strengthen your core.

10) Warrior Pose II (Veerbhadrasana)

Instructions to practice this pose:

Step-1: Stand with your feet together and hands by your side.

Step-2: Now extend your right leg and keep your left hand extended backward.

Step-3: **Now slowly and gently** bend your right knee so that you get into the lunge position.

Step-4: After that twist your torso to face your bent right leg.

Step-5: Now slightly turn your left foot sideways about 40 to 60 degrees to give you that extra support.

Step-6: Start exhaling and straighten your arms and raise your body up and away from your bent knee.

Step-7: Stretch your arms upwards and slowly tilt your torso backwards so your back forms and arch.

Step-8: Now in the end of this pose exhale and straighten your right knee. Now push off your right leg and come back to your initial position. You can use your hands to support you. Do not rush out of this pose; you might injure your back or legs.

Step-9: Repeat this pose for the other leg as well.

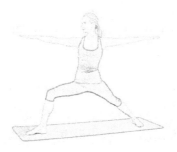

Fig. 1.10 Warrior Pose II

Precautions:

1. If you are suffering from high blood pressure or back trouble please avoid this pose.

Other benefits:

1. This pose stretches your back, strengthens your thighs.

2. This pose also strengths your buttocks.

Chapter 12: The Benefits Of Yoga

The numerous beneficial effects of different yoga techniques include improved body flexibility, stress reduction, boosted performance and achievement of inner peace and self-realization. The yoga techniques has been promoted as complementary treatment strategy to help in the treatment or various diseases such as asthma, anxiety disorders, depression, coronary heart problems as well as extensive rehabilitation for illnesses such as traumatic brain injury and musculoskeletal problems. The techniques of yoga have also been recommended as behavioral treatment for substance abuse (such as alcohol and drug abuse) and smoking cessation.

If you attend yoga classes, you may take advantage of the following benefits:

Spiritual

Contentment

Tranquility and inner peace

Life with direction, purpose and meaning

Mental

Intellectual enhancement, which leads to and enhanced decision-making skills

Relief and prevention from stress-associated disorders

Relief of stress brought about by successful emotional control

Physical

Improved immune system

Increased energy levels

Weight control

Relaxation of muscular strength

Improved abdominal strength

Improved digestion

Improved cardiovascular endurance

Improved balance and body flexibility

At this point, a word of caution with regard to the inappropriate practice of yoga is necessary. With the endless advantages may come injury for beginners or those individuals who practice it without adequate instruction. More than 18 million Americans around the world are reported to employ some form of yoga and medical experts as well as health care providers are recording injuries such as cartilage tears; back and neck pains; and ligament and muscle sprains.

Yoga societies recommend at least 100 hours of training under the supervision of a yoga experts. About 5,000 yoga instructors all over the world reportedly have satisfied that requirement. Before attending a particular yoga class, inquire about the training and credentials of the yoga instructor. Before committing yourself to a set program, you may wish to sit on a class and observe first.

Yoga for Specific Health Problems

Multiple sclerosis – According to experts from the Oregon Health and Science University, some type of yoga forms may help lessen fatigue in individuals suffering from multiple sclerosis (MS). These experts have employed the Iyengar form of yoga for individuals suffering from MS.

Rheumatoid Arthritis – 1.3 million of Americans are reported to be suffering from rheumatoid arthritis. 75 percent of this population is women. Yoga may be beneficial for people suffering from arthritis for pain and stiffness relief, improvement of the range of motion and boost strength for everyday activities.

Individuals who are elderly or inactive – if you love a sedentary lifestyle, yoga may be the most suitable exercise for both the body and mind to start your active life. Yoga also helps to lessen stress in addition to improving the posture and strengthening the muscles and bones. Since you really do not have to be at the optimum physical shape in order to do yoga, it is the most ideal activity for inactive people as well as for the elderly who might not otherwise engage in exercise.

Ongoing Research on the Benefits of Yoga

The National Institutes of Health is currently assessing yoga as an alternative treatment for insomnia, chronic lower back pain and other disorders.

CHAPTER 13: TIPS FOR A YOGA NEWBIE

Regardless if you are just starting with yoga at home or in a class and instructor, you can learn the basics of yoga in various ways. A good instructor is always the first bet of course but if it's not possible, there are several yoga books, training videos, audio tapes, CD and DVD and websites you can learn and understand yoga. Likewise, there are a host of Yoga teachers offering classes in offices, halls, private studios and even schools that aim to cater the needs of both sexes. Yoga classes are also available now online. And because yoga can be demanding, you must further understand its principles as well as your body's ability.

- Yoga can be energizing, slow or gentle, invigorating, technical or demanding or most of the times, a combination of these qualities. Each style has its own methods and takes on philosophy and practitioners can base their preferences on it.

- As a beginner, you may practice yoga for at least 15-20 minutes in your first week. As you progress, you can do it for 30-40 minutes and learn new poses. Increase your duration later on to 1 1/2 hours for best results.

- You can practice yoga at anytime of the day that is convenient for you but you should not have eaten any foods for at least 3 hours. Preferably, do it at the same time each day so it will become a habit.

- Practicing yoga in the morning and evening is better so there will be fewer distractions especially if you are doing it at home. Doing it in the morning will keep you energetic and alert for the entire day's activities. If you'll do it in the evening, it helps you reduce stress, feel relax and calm the mind that promotes a good night sleep.

- Doing it a home with the help of instructional CDs or online will give you the chance to do it with family and group of friends. If you prefer doing it in a studio, you can work with other students and learn new tips and poses with the help of a teacher.

- It is ideal to practice yoga in open spaces such as balcony or terrace. If doing it in a room, make sure that it is free from clutter and furniture, free from noise and with fresh air for more comfort.

- For beginners, the most important focus is mastering the poses while breathing correctly. This sounds simple to others but it takes more concentration to keep aware of the positions of the arms, core, back, legs, hands, feet and head while breathing deeply.

- Practicing yoga poses is considered an exercise and doing it improperly may lead to injury. You should have a clear sense of what are your limits and the right pace to master every pose.

- Moreover, yoga isn't a competition so take your time to master every poses. Listen to your body - pain and tightness means you need to warm up more, skip a day of practice or modify your pose. A thorough warm-up is ideal so look for a class that has it.

- Before joining any kind of activity or exercise, better to consult your doctor first to determine any medical condition that might be compromised in safely practicing yoga.

- Wear clothes that are comfortable and not too tight so you can gracefully perform the poses without yanking up your shirt or minding your baggy pants and getting conscious on how you look.

- Although water is not necessary for most yoga classes (except from hot yoga), still come hydrated. Don't eat at least for 2 hours before you practice as bendy shapes can affect how you feel in the inside.

- Yoga isn't just about those bendy shapes but it's about being fit and strong. It is about being in the present by listening to our own breath. Likewise, never push too much into pain. If it doesn't feel right or it hurts you, tell the teacher. Be truthful to your body and how it feels. You may want to be gentle and kind to yourself and not abuse your body.

- Don't mind other people in the room during the practice. They don't really care how you look, what are you wearing or if you look funny doing a pose. Focus on your breathing. Your mind should be steer clear of foreign thoughts or else, you will never do the poses successfully. Listen to your breathe and be present at the moment.

- Whilst there can be talk about the Divine or God, yoga is not a type of religion. It doesn't force you to believe in anything but it's about the experience. Learn the postures, practice breathing, meditate and give yourself a treat by harvesting the benefits it offers. Yoga is also a tool to enhance whatever your religious beliefs are through body-mind awareness.

- Concentrate and be conscientious on what you are doing on your mat. Don't talk while exercising and focus on your position and breathe. If possible stay away from all distractions especially if you're doing it at home.

- Your breathing is an important aspect of yoga. Breathe deeply and slowly and use your nose breathing in and out.

- Never practice yoga if you are under the influence of alcohol. Likewise, you don't have to totally give up smoking or become a vegetarian before you start practicing yoga. Yoga can aid you to overcome those bad habits and bring alignment in your spiritual aspect to overcome those vices you wanted to get rid of.

- be mindful of the space around you as yoga classes tend to be packed out. Leave enough space for other students and yourself. Respect and be aware of the space to avoid injuries as well when you topple from a certain pose.

- You must invest on a good mat. Whilst plastic vinyl and PVC are widely use in most yoga mats, there are new and safe options flourishing the marketplace. There are yoga mats made of dried grass, natural rubber, organic cotton and biodegradable compounds. Whatever your preference is, invest in purchasing a good mat since it is the most important tool you'll use during class.

Do not feel bad if the instructor or teacher will correct you as it is the best way for you to learn. Avoid judging yourself as well or compare to what other students are doing. Keep thing light-hearted and enjoy yourself on the mat. It is an individual process so trust your own judgement on what you can do. Over time, you will get to know the difference of being afraid to do something over what is impossible or harmful to do. There's no need to rush as your body knows its limit and capacity.

Why Practice Yoga

Yoga is good for our cardiovascular health. It also develops strength and flexibility as well as mental clarity and emotional balance. This is safe for all ages and even those with injuries or sick can modify yoga to suit them. It initiates healing from within and a good way to create wellness. Moreover, it is a form of practice that will give you overall benefits: strength, flexibility, balance, endurance and relaxation. Hence, the ultimate challenge of the body and mind.

The different positions in yoga exercise our different ligaments and tendons. If you live a sedentary life, yoga can help you become flexible. You can attained it easily specifically on parts that that are not consciously worked out in other types of activity.

More than just exercising our joints, stretching our body and releasing our tensions, yoga can also massage our internal organs in a thorough manner. It massages and stimulate the organs in a wholesome way especially those that are hardly stimulated such as the prostate. This act provides nourishment while flushing out toxins out of the body.

Nonetheless, yoga is an overall health and fitness practice that not only targets our physical aspects but also touches our spiritual and mental areas. Through meditation, we can all harmonize our mind and body. It helps achieve an emotional balance by creating conditions that would make us unaffected in our surroundings. In turn, we will be able to develop positive outlook in life.

CHAPTER 14: YOGA POSES FOR WEIGHT LOSS

There are many poses that can help with weight loss, toning and muscle building. The following are just a few of many.

The Warrior Pose

This pose is "one of the best yoga poses for weightless" and promotes strengthening and toning in the arms, shoulders, back, and legs. If you have back or neck issues this pose will allow for a great stretch and help release tension. Here's how to do it:

Start in a standing position with your feet shoulder width apart. Take a big step forward, allowing your heel of the back foot rise off the floor, your toes remaining on the mat.

Now, slowly bring your arms up, palms facing each other. Make sure you look up towards the ceiling but don't hurt your neck.

When you are at this stage, you should feel a slight pull in your back and hind leg.

Hold this pose for several slow breaths, and slowly come out of it in the reverse that you went into it.

When you remember your poses and know what you like to do next, you will get better at going pose-to-pose more smoothly. You should repeat this pose two to three times on each side.

The Chair Pose

The chair pose is on that is great for your thighs and glutes. It is also wonderful for the back, hips, ankles, and knees. To perform this pose, you simply have to follow these steps:

Begin by standing with your feet together. As you inhale, raise your hands above your head.

Stretch your arms above your head as you exhale, and bend your knees as you inhale once again.

Your back should be straight and your backside should be slightly protruded.

Holding this pose for about 60 seconds is ideal, however, it may be difficult at first. Of course, you can work your way into it, starting with just 20 seconds and then 30, then 40 and so on until you are able to stay there for about 60 seconds or more.

The Bridge Pose

The bridge pose is said to have amazing flat tummy powers. It is also said to help tone the arms and legs, as well as aiding digestion and kidney function. It's quite simple to do.

First, you simply lie down on your back with your feet together and your hands at your sides, relaxed.

Now, as you exhale, slowly bring your back and chest towards the ceiling. Stretch your hands toward your feet.

You should feel a good stretch in your abdomen and lower belly. Also, you should make sure you are breathing normally.

On the exhale bring your chest and back down.

You can make this move a little harder just by simply raising one leg when you carry out the pose. This will add a little more pressure to the supporting leg, as it adds more body weight. Make sure that you do both legs to create balance.

The Locust Pose

This pose is one of the 12 basic yoga postures and is considered one of the best for weight loss. Here's how you do it!

You can start by lying down on your belly with your face down and your palms facing the floor.

When you inhale, lift your legs—without bending your knees—and bring your chest off the ground as well.

You should feel a nice stretch in the abdominal and calf areas.

A good way to think of this exercise is to balance on your belly.

You can hold this position for about 10 to 20 seconds at a time. Do this two to three times.

This exercise is meant to target fat on the thighs and belly as well as provide a gentle stretch to the back, arms, and legs. The locust pose was also meant to increase flexibility

The Plank

The plank is a very well known exercise, but many people do not know that it actually comes from yoga! It may be one of the best exercises you could do to strengthen your core. Once you hold a plank for a minute and do it regularly, you won't be long building muscles in your arms and abdomen. Perform the following steps to get this plank move down like a pro!

Begin on your hands and knees. From here, you can simply out stretch your legs.

Now you should be in a pre-pushup position. Now hold yourself there

You can hold this position for as long as you feel you can. It is a more difficult exercise, so doing it for 20 to 30 seconds would be a good goal in the beginning.

Fun fact: the longest plank hold in the world was a total of eight hours and one minute, by Mao Weidong in 2016. Imagine how strong this man is!

The Triangle Pose

This pose may not leave you shaking or feeling weak, like the plank does, but it will help sculpt your abs and allow for a nice, gentle stretch in the side and legs. Due to the soft twist that this pose provides, it also aids in digestion and help reduce belly fat.

First, you stand with your legs in a wide stance. Let your arms fall to your sides in a relaxed manner.

As you inhale, raise your arms to a 90-degree angle. Now, as you exhale, bend at the hip to whichever side you feel more comfortable with.

Reach your hand to your foot. And let the other arm stay at a 90-degree angle to your body—but in the air, towards the sky.

You can hold this position for around six to seven breaths.

Make sure to do the same with the other side, as well.

The Downward Dog

The downward dog is used to rest the body and at the same time tone the arms. This pose is also wonderful for those who have any back or back related leg problems, as this pose provides a good stretch to the back and legs.

Begin on your hands and knees. When you inhale, extend your legs, balancing on your toes and pull your pelvis up into the air.

Extend your arms, locking your elbows and make sure that your palms are flat on the floor. Your feet should also be flat to the floor, now.

During the time that you hold this position, you should be pushing your weight onto your hands and feet.

It is important to breathe while you are doing these exercises. When you do not breathe enough or correctly, you could end up getting dizzy. So taking deep breaths and focusing on your breathing should carry you through this exercise.

The Upward Dog or "Sun Salutations"

You can go right from downward dog to the upward dog (sun salutations). This is a great warm up exercise. It provides a soft stretch to the belly and arms and is said to "build internal heat." This helps quicken the metabolism and tone the muscles that are being stretched. The exercise is also said to "trim your waist!" Who doesn't want a tiny waist?

Going from the Downward Dog

As said earlier, you can go right from the downward dog to this pose. Many people like to do this, as it increases arms and chest strength as well as provide stretches to similar places.

Right from step three of the downward dog, breathe out and begin to lower yourself to the ground.

Once you are in something similar to a plank position, begin to arch your back and bring your chest up to the ceiling.

Make sure that—just like in the downward dog—you are pushing your weight into your hands.

When you carry out these steps, it is important to make sure that the top of your foot (the opposite of the sole of your feet) should be flat to the ground. This is a little difficult to explain, so finding a picture on the internet may be more helpful.

The Upward Dog by Itself

You can do the upward dog by itself. Simply begin in a plank-like position and lower your pelvis to the ground, flattening out your feet. You can now follow the steps we discussed previously.

The Half Moon Pose

This pose is especially good for your glutes and legs. It also provides a good deep sketch in the back and side. Many people find that if they have a back injury or high blood pressure, this move is not good for them. Despite this, people find that the half moon pose can help with back problems, as it moves and twists and spine. To do it, follow these steps:

Start with your feet together, and raise your hands above your head, palms together.

Now, as you exhale, slowly bend your torso to the left (or right)—making sure that your hands stay above your head. They should point in the direction that you are bending.

You should feel a stretch on your opposite side. However, if you feel any ripping or tearing, you should stop immediately and apply heat.

As you inhale, now, come back up to a standing position. Make sure you do the other side, as well.

Of course, these are just some of the moves that you can carry out to lose weight. To maximize your chances of losing weight and toning your body you should be eating healthy, exercising and making certain lifestyle changes along with yoga. All of these things together should help you lose weight quite quickly if you stick with it.

CHAPTER 15: MOUNTAIN POSE

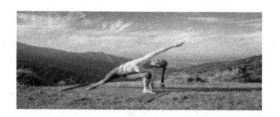

Mountain Pose ('Tadasana') is the basic standing pose that forms the basis for other standing asanas. Stand with your feet parallel and shoulder-width apart. Inhale, lift your toes from the mat, spread them apart as wide as you can, and then lower them back down to the ground. Try to distribute your weight evenly across both feet. Take care that you are not leaning in any particular direction. Aim to emulate the stability of a mountain, from which this pose takes its name.

Take another breath. As you inhale, contract the muscles around your kneecaps and thighs. Position your pelvis so that your hips are aligned with your ankles. Do not stiffen or lock your knees - your aim should be to stand with your legs straight but not rigid. Inhale again, this time stretching out your torso and lengthening your spine. Imagine that the top of your head is being drawn up to the ceiling.

Push your chest out as you exhale, drop your shoulders and point your hands towards the mat. Take another breath and this time, as you breath in, lift your arms into the air and clasp your hands together above your head. Continue to breathe deeply and extend through your arms, hands and fingers. Remain in this pose for 2-3 minutes. Exhale and smoothly release your arms from their position, bringing them to rest by your sides once more.

Chair Pose

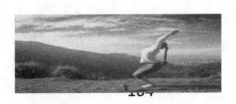

Chair Pose ('Utkatasana') is great for developing your balance, strengthening your back, working your abdominal muscles and toning your thighs.

Start in Mountain Pose, as outlined in the previous section. Your hands should be clasped together above your head. If you do not find it comfortable to have your hands clasped together, it is fine to keep your palms pressed firmly together instead. Take a deep breath and as you exhale, bend your knees. Aim to make your thighs parallel to the floor. The front of your body should be approximately at a right angle to your thighs. Keep your thighs in alignment.

Expand your shoulders, holding them relaxed but firm. Keep your back lengthened - no hunching or rounding! After remaining in this position for 30-60 seconds, exhale and straighten your knees, bringing your arms down to a relaxed position by your sides.

Camel Pose

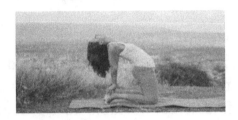

Also known as 'Ushtraasana,' Camel Pose provides you with a great opportunity to stretch the muscles in your back, shoulders and arms. This is not a pose to open your practice with - start with a few easier asanas first to warm up your muscles first.

Get on your knees, keeping your calves flat against the ground. Your heels should be against your buttocks. Gently reach around and hold your right and left ankles in your right and left hands respectively. Take a deep breath. As you inhale, push your abdomen forward, lift your buttocks from your heels and arch your back. Breathe steadily as you hold this position for 1-3 minutes. Exhale and slowly return to your original kneeling position.

Take care not to tense your neck. Aim to keep your muscles soft and relaxed at all times. Never force your neck and shoulders into a position that feels very uncomfortable or unnatural.

If you are not yet flexible enough to maintain a hold on your ankles or feet whilst in this pose, use tall foam blocks instead. Place a block next to each foot and instead of holding onto your ankles, rest your hands on the blocks.

Downward-Facing Dog

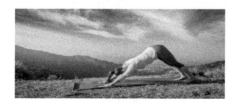

Downward-Facing Dog Pose ('Adhomukhasvanasana') is so named because in performing this asana you emulate the way in which a dog stretches when it wakes from a nap. Downward-Facing Dog is good for enhancing general flexibility and strength. It provides a great stretch for your calves. It enhances circulation and can be a good quick remedy for tiredness.

Begin by getting on the floor and positioning yourself on your hands and knees. Keep your knees beneath your hipbones and your hands an inch or two in front of your shoulders. Keep your fingers spread. Lift and turn your toes under. Take a deep breath and then as you exhale, move your knees upwards and away from the floor. Do not attempt to push your heels down to the ground just yet.

Push your coccyx and pelvis towards the ceiling, and contract the muscles in your thighs. With your next exhalation, push your heels down to the floor and straighten your knees. However, do not lock or stiffen them! Contract the outer muscles of your arms and press your fingers down into the floor. Widen your shoulder blades. Do not allow your head to hang between your arms; hold your head aligned between your upper arms.

Hold this asana for 2-3 minutes. When you have finished, exhale and gently bend your knees as you come out of the pose.

Life throws many curveballs our way; this often makes it difficult to stay happy all the time; still, a life devoid of happiness, is meaningless. By practicing yoga, you can easily improve your state of well-being and happiness, and restore tranquility and joy back into your life. Below are a few great poses that can help you become happy and amplify your happiness.

Goddess Pose

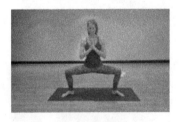

The goddess pose, or utkatakonasana, is one of the most effectivehappiness inducing yoga poses. The goddess pose is an empowering and energizing pose that stretches your chest, groin, and hips, helps you lose weight, improves blood circulation, and augments the serotonin levels in your body, consequently improving your mood.

How to Perform It

1. To perform this pose, first enter the mountain pose.

2. Now, stand up and keep your arms at the sides.

3. Place your hands on the hips. Turn towards the right and step both feet about four feet apart. Slightly turn the toes outwards, exhale and bend the knees over the toes.

4. Lower the hips and enter the squat position. Try bringing your hips as parallel as possible to the floor.

5. Extend the arms towards the sides and keep the palms faced downwards. Spiral

the thumbs upwards towards the roof and move the palms forward.

6. Bend the elbows and then point the fingertips towards the roof. Keep your forearms and upper arms at a 90-degree angle.

7. Tuck the tailbone in lightly. Press the buttocks forward and keep the knees and toes aligned. Hold for ten breaths.

8. Slowly, return the hands to your buttocks and keep the spine upright. Straighten the legs and step back your feet together. Relax and take a few deep breaths.

Practice this pose for five to ten minutes daily to escalate your happiness level

Adho Mukha Savanasana

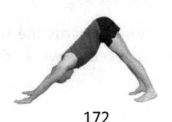

Downward Facing Dog, also known as adho mukha savanasana, is an excellent pose for curbing unnecessary and incessant mood swings and changing gloominess into happiness. In addition, it improves bone density, enhances blood circulation, eliminates back pain, stiffness, and increases your flexibility.

How to Perform It

1. Begin on all fours. Your hands should be beneath your shoulders and the palms should press onto the floor.

2. Tuck the toes under. Now, slowly lift the knees off the ground as you gently straighten the legs.

3. Maintain the pose for five to ten breaths. Practice it daily to elevate your mood and stay happy.

In addition to the above poses, the surya namaskar also improves your mental well-being and reduces mood swings.

CHAPTER 17: SAFETY AND PRECAUTION TIPS

Yoga is a rigorous exercise so you need to make sure that you put your safety first. Here are some of the helpful safety tips that will help keep you safe when practicing yoga:

1.Wear comfortable clothes

If you want to reap the optimum benefits of yoga then you have to wear loose and comfortable clothes. This will allow you to move easily and do the poses accurately. You can wear a tank top and even wear leggings or jogging pants.

2.Know your limits.

Yoga can be challenging to some. It is important that you know what your limits are when practicing yoga. Yoga is not a sport so there's no need to compete with others. Do the poses at your own pace. To avoid any injuries it is important to determine what poses you can and cannot do. If you are in pain then you need to stop.

3.Rest in between poses.

You have to listen to your body. If you feel tired or uncomfortable then take time to rest. Resting between poses is necessary- especially if you are a beginner.

4.Use a yoga mat.

It is important to use a yoga mat when you are doing the poses. You can also use a pillow if you feel uncomfortable doing some of the poses.

5.Do warm up exercises.

Yoga classes usually incorporate several warm up exercises. However, if you are doing it at home it is best to come up with your own warm up exercises. You can do basic stretching exercises before doing a certain yoga sequence.

6.See your doctor when needed.

If you are suffering from a disease or you are recovering from a serious injury then it is best to ask your doctor if it is safe for you to do yoga. If you feel persistent muscle pains consult your doctor.

Yoga is a great exercise that you can do with your family and friends. Remember that yoga is not a competition so it is okay not to get the poses right during your first few tries.

CONCLUSION

To get started, the best way to do it is to release all expectations and just look at what the full spectrum gets you. You have already done that by reading this book. It is as comprehensive an overview as you are going to get, but it doesn't teach you everything. That is for you to experience on your own.

Look into Yoga Asana classes. Numerous studios offer this, depending on where you are located. Find a studio that hosts trained instructors. Body posture and movements are not to be taken lightly. Those who are not trained, will not know how to direct your movement based on your body type and size. They may end up being injurious to your musculature.

Yoga masters who know what they are doing are certified and have a special demeanor about them. Most of them are at such peace with themselves, that you instantly fall into peace in their presence.

If you can find an instructor who has this, sign up.

The studio that you choose must be peaceful and foster harmonious vibes so that you can feel the peace when you get there. Choose a day to practice Yoga where you are not rushing or stressed to get there. Pick a day when you have no pressing obligations and don't need to rush from one move to the next just so that you can get back to start dinner.

Alter your reading habits for the day that you do your Yoga. It does not have to be spiritual in nature but it has to be positive in spirit. Stay away for the news and things that will frustrate you more than embrace you.

Once you get all these lined up, make it a practice to never miss your Yoga day, and then keep two or three other days of the week where you practice what you have learned in the privacy of your own home.

Yoga is not Pilates or aerobics. It is not Karate or Judo. It is not a class that you do at the studio then forget about until your next session. Yoga is a holistic practice that offers you the tools to engage with the Universe. Treat it as such. If you choose to do Yoga for its health benefits, its breathing improvement, and its posture realignment, there is nothing wrong with that. Just remember that other people around you may be looking for more. There is nothing wrong when each of you keeps to his or her own lane. They do not need to tell you that you should go for more, and you shouldn't tell them that they should do less.

What you should do is keep it at the back of your mind that Yoga has the eight limbs that we discussed and that it is available to you at any time, at your own pace, in the privacy of your mind. The eight limbs of Yoga are not something that you need to race through. Take it as it comes. We are all built differently and have a different purpose.

Above all else, keep an open mind and approach it like a new experience. Our bodies, after all, are adept at experiencing new things and this will be something new that your mind and body will enjoy thoroughly. At the very least, that would be the experience to get out of this. And when you come to the end of that line, you find you want to take it one step further, then so be it. Take it as it comes and you will realize that you can find peace as long as you are in search of it.

CPSIA information can be obtained
at www.ICGtesting.com
Printed in the USA
BVHW071001130820
586318BV00013B/1216